The Anatomy of Sports Injuries

Your Illustrated Guide to Prevention, Diagnosis and Treatment

Second Edition

Brad Walker

lotus
publishing

First published in 2007. This second edition published in 2013 by
Lotus Publishing
Apple Tree Cottage, Inlands Road,
Nutbourne, Chichester, PO18 8RJ

Anatomical Illustrations Amanda Williams
Exercise Illustrations Matt Lambert
Text Design Wendy Craig
Cover Design Jim Wilkie
Printed and Bound in the UK by Bell & Bain Limited

British Library Cataloguing-in-Publication Data
A CIP record for this book is available from the British Library
ISBN 978 1 905367 38 2

The Library of Congress Cataloguing-in-Publication has catalogued the first edition as follows:
Walker, Brad, 1971-
The anatomy of sports injuries / Brad Walker.
    p. ; cm.
Includes bibliographical references and index.
ISBN 978-1-55643-666-6 (North Atlantic Books : pbk.)
1. Sports injuries--Atlases. I. Title.
[DNLM: 1. Athletic Injuries--Atlases. 2. Athletic Injuries--Handbooks.
3. Athletic Injuries--therapy--Atlases. 4. Athletic
Injuries--therapy--Handbooks. QT 29 W177a 2007]
RD97.W35 2007
617.1′027--dc22
                          2007010564

Contents

Introduction

As sports participation rates increase, so does the occurrence of sport-related injury. As a consequence, there is a need for detailed, easy-to-understand reference books on the prevention, treatment and management of sports injury.

Whilst there are many books dealing with this subject, very few present detailed anatomical information in a way that is easy to understand for everyone from the weekend warrior to the professional athlete; from the first-year personal trainer to the seasoned sports coach or from the recent university graduate to the accomplished sports doctor.

Combining real-life practical experience with detailed theory, Brad Walker presents complex prevention, treatment and management strategies in a way that everyone can understand. Full-colour illustrations provide a visual aid to the workings of the human body during the sports injury management process. The expert yet easy-to-follow information will help the reader prevent sports injury, and in the event that an injury does occur help to treat it effectively, allowing a return to activity in as little time as possible.

The Anatomy of Sports Injuries looks at sport-related injury from every angle. Chapter 1 introduces the concept of sports injury. It explains the different classifications and grades of sports injury and describes the structures and tissues involved. In Chapter 2 key prevention strategies are explained to help reduce the occurrence of sport-related injury. In Chapter 3 a comprehensive treatment and rehabilitation process is outlined to ensure a quick and complete recovery.

Chapters 4–17 provide a detailed overview of 120 sports injuries in an easy-to-locate format. Divided into key areas of the body, each sports injury is described by: the anatomy and physiology involved, possible causes, signs and symptoms, complications, immediate treatment, rehabilitation procedures and long-term prognosis.

Aimed at fitness enthusiasts and health-care professionals of all levels, The Anatomy of Sports Injuries also provides strength and flexibility exercises to aid with sports injury prevention, treatment and rehabilitation. These exercises are by no means exhaustive and merely provide guidance. Consult a healthcare professional for a tailor-made programme to suit your individual needs.

Anatomical Directions

Abduction . . . . A movement away from the midline (of the body or foot/hand).
Adduction . . . . A movement toward the midline (of the body or foot/hand).
Anatomical position . The body is upright with the palms of the hands turned forward.
Anterior . . . . Toward the front of the body (as opposed to posterior).

Circumduction . . . . . Movement in which the distal end of a bone moves in a circle while the
proximal end remains stable.
Contralateral . . . . On the opposite side.
Coronal plane . . . . . . A vertical plane at right angles to the sagittal plane which divides the
body in to anterior and posterior portions.

Deep . . . . Away from the surface (as opposed to superficial).
Depression . . . . Movement of a body part downward.
Distal . . . . Away from the point of origin of a structure (as opposed to proximal).
Dorsal . . . . Relating to the back or posterior portion (as opposed to ventral).

Elevation . . . . Movement of a part of the body upward in the coronal plane.
Eversion . . . . To turn the sole of the foot outward.
Extension . . . . A movement at a joint resulting in separation of two ventral surfaces (as
opposed to flexion).

Flexion . . . . A movement at a joint resulting in approximation of two ventral surfaces
(as opposed to extension).

Horizontal plane . . . A transverse plane at right angle to the long axis of the body.

Inferior . . . . Below or furthest away from the head.
Inversion . . . . To turn the sole of the foot inward.

Lateral . . . . Away from the midline of the body or organ (opposite to medial).

Medial . . . . Toward the midline of the body or organ (opposite to lateral).
Median . . . . Centrally located, situated in the middle of the body.

Opposition . . . . A movement specific to the saddle joint of the thumb that enables the
thumb to touch the tips of the fingers of the same hand.

Palmar . . . . Anterior surface (palm) of the hand.
Plantar . . . . The sole of the foot.
Posterior . . . . Relating to the back or the dorsal aspect of the body (as opposed to
anterior).
Pronation . . . . To turn the palm of the hand down to face the floor or away from
the anatomical position.
Prone . . . . Position of the body in which the ventral surface faces down (as opposed
to supine).
Protraction . . . . Movement forward in the transverse plane.
Proximal . . . . Closer to the centre of the body or to the point of attachment of a limb.

Retraction . . . . Movement backward in the transverse plane.

Rotation . . . . Movement around a fixed axis.

Sagittal plane . . . . . . A vertical plane extending in an anteroposterior direction dividing the body into equal right and left parts.

Superficial . . . . On or near the surface (as opposed to deep).

Superior . . . . Above or closest to the head.

Supination . . . . To turn the palm of the hand up to face the ceiling or toward the anatomical position.

Supine . . . . Position of the body in which the ventral surface faces up (as opposed to prone).

Ventral . . . . Refers to the anterior part of the body (as opposed to dorsal).

Explanation of Sports Injury

No one doubts the benefits of regular structured exercise: elevated cardiovascular fitness, improved muscular strength and increased flexibility all contribute to an enhanced quality of life. However, one of the very few drawbacks of exercise is an increased susceptibility to sports injury.

While sport and exercise participation rates are increasing (a good thing!) injury rates are also on the rise. In fact the US Consumer Product Safety Commission estimates: "between 1991 and 1998, golf and swimming injuries increased 110 percent; ice hockey and weightlifting injuries, 75 percent; soccer injuries, 55 percent; bicycling, 45 percent; volleyball, 44 percent; and football 43 percent" (*Consumer Product Safety Review, 2000*).

WHAT CONSTITUTES A SPORTS INJURY?

Physical injury generally can be defined as any stress on the body that prevents the organism from functioning properly and results in the body employing a process of repair. A sports injury can be further defined as any kind of injury, pain or physical damage that occurs as a result of sport, exercise or athletic activity.

Although the term sports injury can be used to define any trauma sustained as a result of sport and exercise, it usually describes injuries that affect the musculoskeletal system. More serious injuries, such as head, neck and spinal cord trauma, are usually considered separate to common sports injuries like sprains, strains, fractures and contusions.

WHAT IS AFFECTED IN A SPORTS INJURY?

Sports injuries are most commonly associated with the musculoskeletal system, which includes the muscles, bones, joints and associated tissues such as ligaments and tendons. Below is a brief explanation of the components that make up the musculoskeletal system.

Muscles

Muscle is composed of 75% water, 20% protein and 5% mineral salts, glycogen and fat. There are three types of muscle: skeletal, cardiac and smooth. The type of muscle involved with movement is skeletal (also referred to as striated, somatic or voluntary). Skeletal (somatic or voluntary) muscles make up approximately 40% of the total human body weight. Skeletal muscles are under voluntary control, and attach to, and cover over, the bony skeleton. They are capable of powerful, rapid contractions and longer, sustained contractions. Skeletal muscles enable us to perform both feats of strength and controlled, fine movements. They are attached to bone by tendons. The place where a muscle attaches to a relatively stationary point on a bone, either directly or via a tendon, is called the origin. When the muscle contracts, it transmits tension to the bones across one or more joints and movement occurs. The end of the muscle that attaches to the bone that moves is called the insertion.

EXPLANATION OF SPORTS INJURY

Overview of Skeletal Muscle Structure

The functional unit of skeletal muscle is known as a muscle fibre, which is an elongated, cylindrical cell with multiple nuclei, ranging from 10–100 microns in width, and a few millimetres to 30+ centimetres in length. The cytoplasm of the fibre is called the sarcoplasm, which is encapsulated inside a cell membrane called the sarcolemma. A delicate membrane known as the endomysium surrounds each individual fibre.

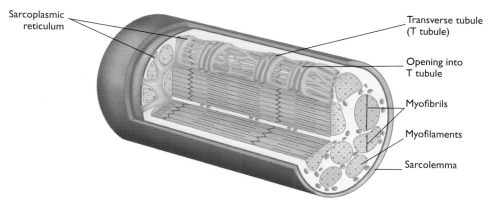

Each skeletal muscle fibre is a single cylindrical muscle cell.

Muscle fibres are grouped together in bundles covered by the perimysium. These bundles are themselves grouped together, and the whole muscle is encased in a sheath called the epimysium. These muscle membranes run through the entire length of the muscle, from the tendon of origin to the tendon of insertion. This whole structure is sometimes referred to as the musculo-tendinous unit.

> NOTE: *As they contract, all muscle types generate heat, and this heat is vitally important in maintaining a normal body temperature. It is estimated that 85% of all body heat is generated by muscle contractions.*

Major muscles include the quadriceps of the thigh and the biceps brachii of the upper arm.

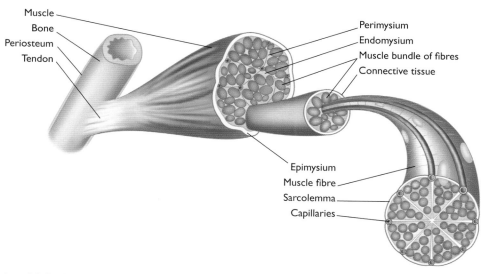

Cross-section of skeletal muscle tissue.

Bones

We are born with approximately 350 bones, but gradually they fuse together until by puberty we have only 206. Bones form the supporting structure of the body and are collectively known as the endoskeleton. (The exoskeleton is well developed in many invertebrates but exists in humans only as teeth, nails and hair). Fully developed bone is the hardest tissue in the body and is composed of 20% water, 30–40% organic matter and 40–50% inorganic matter.

Bone Development and Growth

The majority of bone is formed from a foundation of cartilage, which becomes calcified and then ossified to form true bone. This process occurs through the following four stages:

1. Bone building cells called osteoblasts become active during the second or third month of embryonic life.
2. Initially, the osteoblasts manufacture a matrix of material between the cells, which is rich in a fibrous protein called collagen. This collagen strengthens the tissue. Enzymes then enable calcium compounds to be deposited within the matrix.
3. This intercellular material hardens around the cells, which become osteocytes, living cells that maintain the bone but do not produce new bone.
4. Other cells called osteoclasts break down, remodel and repair bone. This process continues throughout life but slows down with advancing age. Consequently, the bones of elderly people are weaker and more fragile.

In brief, osteoblasts and osteoclasts are the cells that lay down and break down bone respectively, enabling bones to very slowly adapt in shape and strength according to need.

Bone cells sit in cavities called lacunae (singular: lacuna) surrounded by circular layers of very hard matrix that contains calcium salts and larger amounts of collagen fibres. Bones protect internal organs and facilitate movement. Together they form a rigid structure called the skeleton. Major bones include the femur in the thigh and the humerus in the upper arm.

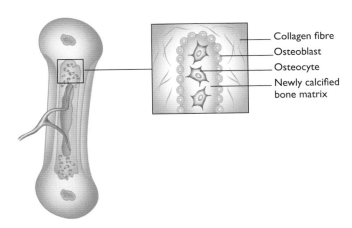

Collagen fibre
Osteoblast
Osteocyte
Newly calcified
bone matrix

Bone development and growth.

Types of Bone According to Density

Compact Bone

Compact bone is dense and looks smooth to the naked eye. Through the microscope, compact bone appears as an aggregation of Haversian systems called osteons. Each system is an elongated cylinder oriented along the long axis of the bone, consisting of a central Haversian canal containing blood vessels, lymph vessels and nerves surrounded by concentric plates of bone called lamellae. In other words, each Haversian system is a group of hollow tubes of bone matrix (lamellae) placed one inside the next. Between these lamellae there are spaces (lacunae) that contain lymph and osteocytes. The lacunae are linked via hair-like canals called canaliculi to the lymph vessels in the Haversian canal, enabling the osteocytes to obtain nourishment from the lymph. This tubular array of lamellae gives great strength to bone.

Other canals called perforating, or Volkmann's, canals run at right angles to the long axis of the bone, connecting the blood vessels and nerve supply within the bone to the periosteum.

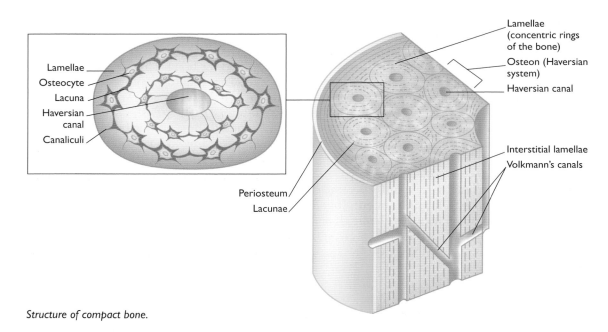

Structure of compact bone.

Spongy Bone (Cancellous Bone)

Spongy bone is composed of small, needle-like trabeculae (singular: trabecula; literally, 'little beams') containing irregularly arranged lamellae and osteocytes interconnected by canaliculi. There are no Haversian systems but rather lots of open spaces, which can be thought of as large Haversian canals, giving a honeycombed appearance. These spaces are filled with red or yellow marrow and blood vessels.

This structure forms a dynamic lattice capable of gradual alteration through realignment in response to stresses of weight, postural change and muscle tension. Spongy bone is found in the epiphyses of long bones, the bodies of the vertebrae and other bones without cavities.

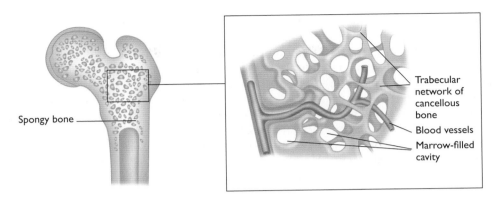

Structure of spongy (cancellous) bone.

Types of Bone According to Shape

Irregular Bones
Irregular bones have complicated shapes; they consist mainly of spongy bone enclosed by thin layers of compact bone. Examples include: some skull bones, the vertebrae and the hip bones.

Flat Bones
Flat bones are thin, flattened bones and are frequently curved; they have a layer of spongy bone sandwiched between two thin layers of compact bone. Examples include: most of the skull bones, the ribs and the sternum.

Short Bones
Short bones are generally cube-shaped; they consist mostly of spongy (cancellous) bone. Examples include: the carpal bones in the wrist and tarsal bones in the ankle.

Sesamoid Bones
From the Latin, meaning 'shaped like a sesame seed', sesamoid bones are a special type of short bone that are formed and embedded within a muscle tendon. Examples are: the patella (kneecap) and the pisiform bone of the wrist.

Long Bones
Long bones are longer than they are wide; they have a shaft with heads at both ends, and consist mostly of compact bone. Examples include: the bones of the limbs, except those of the wrist, hand, ankle and foot (although the bones of the fingers and toes are effectively miniature long bones).

Components of a Long Bone
The transformation of cartilage within a long bone begins at the centre of the shaft. Secondary bone-forming centres develop later, across the ends of the bones. From these growth centres the bone continues to grow through childhood and adolescence, finally ceasing in the early twenties, whereupon the growth regions harden.

Diaphysis
The diaphysis (from Greek, meaning 'a separation') is the shaft or central part of a long bone. It has a marrow-filled cavity (medullary cavity) surrounded by compact bone. It is formed from one or more primary sites of ossification and supplied by one or more nutrient arteries.

Epiphysis

The epiphysis (from Greek, meaning 'excrescence') is the end of a long bone, or any part of a bone separated from the main body of an immature bone by cartilage. It is formed from a secondary site of ossification. It consists largely of spongy bone.

Epiphyseal Line

The epiphyseal line is the remnant of the epiphyseal plate (a flat plate of hyaline cartilage) seen in young, growing bone. The epiphyseal plate is the site of growth of a long bone. By the end of puberty, long bone growth stops and the plate is completely replaced by bone, leaving just the line to mark its previous location.

Articular Cartilage

Articular cartilage is the only remaining evidence of an adult bone's cartilaginous past. It is located where two bones meet (articulate) within a synovial joint. It is smooth, slippery, porous, malleable, insensitive and bloodless. It is massaged by movement, which circulates synovial fluid, oxygen and nutrients.

> NOTE: The degenerative process of osteoarthritis (and the latter stages of some forms of rheumatoid arthritis) involves the breakdown of articular cartilage.

Periosteum

The periosteum is a fibrous connective tissue membrane enveloping the outer surface of bone. It is vascular and provides a highly sensitive, double-layered life support sheath. The outer layer is made up of dense irregular connective tissue. The inner layer, which lies directly against the bone surface, mostly comprises the bone-forming osteoblasts and the bone-destroying osteoclasts.

The periosteum is supplied with nerve fibres, lymphatic vessels and blood vessels that enter the bone through nutrient canals. It is attached to the bone by collagen fibres known as Sharpey's fibres. The periosteum also provides the anchoring point for tendons and ligaments.

Medullary Cavity

The medullary cavity is the cavity of the diaphysis (i.e. the central section of a long bone). It contains marrow: red in the young, turning to yellow in many bones in maturity.

Red Marrow

Red marrow is a red, gelatinous substance composed of red and white blood cells in a variety of developmental forms. Red marrow cavities are typically found within the spongy bone of long bones and flat bones. In adults the red marrow, which creates new red blood cells, occurs only in the head of the femur and the head of the humerus and, much more importantly, in the flat bones such as the sternum and irregular bones such as the hip bones. These are the sites routinely used for obtaining red marrow samples when problems with the blood-forming tissues are suspected.

Yellow Marrow

Yellow marrow is a fatty connective tissue that no longer produces blood cells.

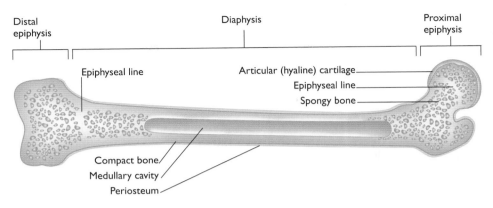

Components of a long bone.

Cartilage

Cartilage is a specialized fibrous connective tissue. Its main purpose is to provide a smooth surface for the movement of joints, and absorb impact and friction when bones bump and rub together. It exists either as a temporary formation that is later replaced by bone, or as a permanent supplementation to bone; it is not as hard or as strong as bone. Cartilage strength comes mainly from the strength of the collagen it contains. Cartilage is relatively non-vascular (not penetrated by blood vessels) and is mainly nourished by surrounding tissue fluids. Types include: hyaline cartilage, fibrocartilage and elastic cartilage.

The most important is hyaline (articular) cartilage, which is made up of collagen fibres and water. Hyaline cartilage forms the temporary foundation of cartilage from which many bones develop, thereafter existing in relation to bone as:

• The articular cartilage of synovial joints.
• Cartilage plates between separately ossifying areas of bone during growth.
• The xiphoid process of the sternum (which ossifies late or not at all) and the costal cartilages.

Hyaline cartilage also exists in the nasal septum, most cartilages of the larynx, and the supporting rings of the trachea and bronchi.

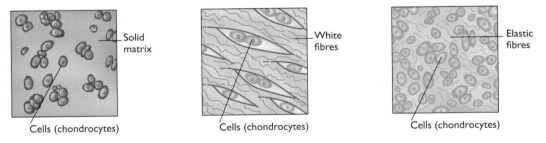

Structure of cartilage; a) hyaline cartilage, b) white fibrocartilage, c) yellow elastic cartilage.

Ligaments

Ligaments are the fibrous connective tissues that connect bone to bone. Composed of dense regular connective tissue, ligaments contain more elastin than tendons and so are more elastic. Ligaments provide stability for the joints and, with the bones, either allow or limit movement of the limbs.

EXPLANATION OF SPORTS INJURY

Tendons

Tendons are the fibrous connective tissues that connect muscle to bone. Their collagen fibres are arranged in a parallel pattern, which enables resistance to high, unidirectional tensile loads when the attached muscle contracts. Tendons work together with muscles to exert force on bones and produce movement.

Joints

Joints (also called articulations) enable movement, giving the rigid bony skeleton mobility. They are also sites where forces are absorbed and transmitted and where growth takes place. There are three main types of joint: fibrous joints, which have very little or no movement; cartilaginous joints, which are either immovable or only slightly movable; and synovial joints, which are freely moveable.

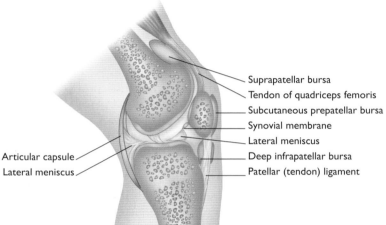

Suprapatellar bursa
Tendon of quadriceps femoris
Subcutaneous prepatellar bursa
Synovial membrane
Lateral meniscus
Deep infrapatellar bursa
Patellar (tendon) ligament

Articular capsule
Lateral meniscus

The knee joint; right leg, mid-sagittal view.

As synovial joints are freely movable, they are the joints most often involved with sports injuries. Major synovial joints include: the knee, hip, shoulder and elbow. Synovial joints share the following features, all of which can be damaged in a sports injury:

Articular capsule

The articular capsule surrounds and envelopes the entire synovial joint. It consists of an outer layer of fibrous tissue and an inner layer, the synovial membrane, which secretes synovial fluid to lubricate and nourish the joint. The joint capsule is strengthened by strong bands of ligament (see above).

Joint cavity

Neither fibrous nor cartilaginous joints have a joint cavity, while synovial joints possess a joint cavity that contains synovial fluid.

Hyaline articular cartilage

Hyaline cartilage covers the end of bones and provides a smooth, slippery surface that allows the joint to move freely. The job of articular cartilage is to reduce friction during movement and absorb shock.

Bursa

A bursa (plural bursae) is a small sac filled with viscid fluid. Bursae are most commonly found at the point in the joint where the muscle and tendon slide across the bone. The job of a bursa is to reduce friction and provide smooth movement for the joint.

The Seven Types of Synovial Joint

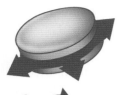

Plane or Gliding
Movement occurs when two generally flat or slightly curved surfaces glide across one another. Examples: the acromioclavicular joint and the intercarpal joints of the wrist.

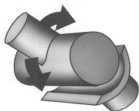

Hinge
Movement occurs around a transverse axis, as in the hinge of the lid of a box. A protrusion of one bone fits into a concave or cylindrical articular surface of another, permitting flexion and extension. Examples: the interphalangeal joints of the digits and the elbow.

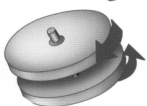

Pivot
Movement takes place around a vertical axis, like the hinge of a gate. A more or less cylindrical articular surface of bone protrudes into and rotates within a ring formed by bone or ligament. Example: the proximal radioulnar joint at the elbow.

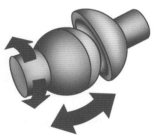

Spheroidal or Ball-and-Socket
Consists of a 'ball' formed by the spherical or hemispherical head of one bone which rotates within the concave 'socket' of another, allowing flexion, extension, adduction, abduction, circumduction and rotation. Thus, they are multi-axial and allow the greatest range of movement of all joints. Examples: the glenohumeral joint and the hip.

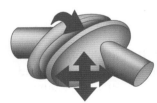

Ellipsoid
Have an ellipsoid articular surface that fits into a matching concavity, which permits flexion, extension and some abduction and adduction. Example: the metacarpophalangeal joints of the hand (but not the thumb).

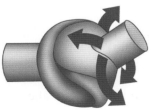

Saddle
Articulating surfaces have convex and concave areas, and so resemble two 'saddles' that accommodate each other's convex to concave surfaces. Similar to ellipsoid joints, they allow flexion, extension, abduction and adduction but more rotational movement, for example, allowing the 'opposition' of the thumb to the fingers. Example: the carpometacarpal joint of the thumb.

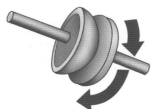

Condylar/bicondylar
Reciprocal convex/concave joint surface(s) allow flexion, extension and limited rotation around a longitudinal axis. Example: the tibiofemoral joint of the knee.

IS THE SPORTS INJURY ACUTE OR CHRONIC?

Regardless of where the injury occurs within the body, or the seriousness of the injury, sports injuries are commonly classified in one of two ways: acute or chronic.

Acute Injuries
These refer to sports injuries that occur in an instant. Common examples of acute injuries are bone fractures, muscle and tendon strains, ligament sprains and contusions. Acute injuries usually result in pain, swelling, tenderness, weakness and the inability to use or place weight on the injured area.

Chronic injuries
These refer to sports injuries that occur over an extended period of time and are sometimes called overuse injuries. Common examples of chronic injuries are tendinitis, bursitis and stress fractures. Chronic injuries, like acute injuries, also result in pain, swelling, tenderness, weakness and the inability to use or place weight on the injured area.

HOW ARE SPORTS INJURIES CLASSIFIED?

As well as classifying a sports injury as acute or chronic, sports injuries are also classified according to their severity. Injuries are graded into one of three classifications: mild, moderate or severe.

Mild
A mild sports injury will result in minimal pain and swelling. It will not adversely affect sporting performance and the affected area is neither tender to touch nor deformed in any way.

Moderate
A moderate sports injury will result in some pain and swelling. It will have a limiting affect on sporting performance and the affected area will be mildly tender to touch. Some discoloration at the injury site may also be present.

Severe
A severe sports injury will result in increased pain and swelling. It will not only affect sporting performance but will also affect normal daily activities. The injury site is usually very tender to touch, and discoloration and deformity are common.

HOW ARE SPRAIN AND STRAIN INJURIES CLASSIFIED?

The term sprain refers to an injury of the ligaments, as opposed to a strain, which refers to an injury of the muscle or tendon. Remember ligaments attach bone to bone, whereas tendons attach muscle to bone.

Injuries to the ligaments, muscles and tendons are usually graded into three categories. These types of injury are referred to as: first-, second- or third-degree sprains and strains.

First-degree
A first-degree sprain/strain is the least severe. It is the result of some minor stretching of the ligaments, muscles or tendons and is accompanied by mild pain, some swelling and joint stiffness. There is usually very little loss of joint stability as a result of a first-degree sprain/strain.

Second-degree
A second-degree sprain/strain is the result of both stretching and some tearing of the ligaments, muscles or tendons. There is increased swelling and pain associated with a second-degree sprain/strain and a moderate loss of stability around the joint.

Third-degree
A third-degree sprain/strain is the most severe of the three. A third-degree sprain/strain is the result of a complete tear or rupture of one or more of the ligaments, muscles or tendons and will result in massive swelling, severe pain and gross instability.

One interesting point to note about a third-degree sprain/strain is that shortly after the injury most of the localized pain may disappear. This is a result of the nerve endings being severed, which causes a lack of feeling at the injury site.

2

Sports Injury Prevention

INTRODUCTION TO SPORTS INJURY PREVENTION

In a recent article titled '*Managing Sports Injuries*', the author estimated that every day more than 27,000 Americans sprain their ankle. On top of this, *Sports Medicine Australia* estimates that 1 in 17 participants in sport and exercise suffer a sports injury playing their favorite sport. This figure is even higher for contact sports like football. However, the truly disturbing fact is that up to 50 per cent of these injuries may have been prevented.

If improving sporting performance is the goal, then there is no better way to do that than by staying injury free. To follow are a number of tips and strategies that will help prevent sports injury. When properly implemented and routinely followed, they have the potential to reduce the incidence of sports injury by up to 50 per cent.

Before moving on, please note that any single injury prevention technique discussed in this chapter is just one component that can help to reduce the overall risk of injury. The best results are achieved when all the techniques are used in combination with each other. When it comes to sports injury, prevention is better than cure.

WARM-UP

Warm-up activities are a crucial part of any exercise or sports training. The importance of a structured warm-up routine should not be underestimated when it comes to the prevention of sports injury.

An effective warm-up has a number of key elements. These elements, or parts, should all work together to minimize the likelihood of sports injury from physical activity.

Warming-up prior to any physical activity has a number of benefits, but its main purpose is to prepare the body and mind for more strenuous activity. One of the ways it achieves this is by helping to increase the body's core temperature while increasing the body's muscle temperature. Increasing muscle temperature will help to make the muscles loose and supple.

An effective warm-up also has the effect of increasing both heart rate and respiratory rate. This increases blood flow, which in turn increases the delivery of oxygen and nutrients to the working muscles. All this helps to prepare the muscles, tendons and joints for more strenuous activity.

How Should the Warm-up Be Structured?

It is important to start the warm-up routine with the easiest and most gentle activity, building upon each part with more energetic activities until the body is at a physical and mental peak. This is the state in which the body is most prepared for the physical activity to come, and where the likelihood of sports injury has been minimized. To achieve these goals, the warm-up should be structured as follows:

There are four key elements, or parts, which should be included to ensure an effective and complete warm-up. They are:

1. The general warm-up
2. Static stretching
3. The sport-specific warm-up
4. Dynamic stretching

All four parts are equally important and any one part should not be neglected or thought of as unnecessary. All four elements work together to bring the body and mind to a physical peak, ensuring the athlete is prepared for the activity to come. This process will help ensure the athlete has a minimal risk of sports injury.

1. General warm-up

The general warm-up should consist of light physical activity. The fitness level of the participating athlete should govern both the intensity (how hard) and duration (how long) of the general warm-up. A general warm-up for the average person should take 5–10 minutes and result in a light sweat.

The aim of the general warm-up is to elevate the heart rate and respiratory rate. This in turn increases the blood flow and helps with the transportation of oxygen and nutrients to the working muscles. It also helps to increase the muscle temperature, allowing for a more effective static stretch.

2. Static stretching

Static stretching is a very safe and effective form of stretching. There is limited risk of injury (when performed correctly) and it is extremely beneficial for overall flexibility. During this part of the warm-up, static stretching should include all the major muscle groups and should last 5–10 minutes.

Static stretching is performed by placing the body in a position whereby the muscle (or group of muscles) to be stretched is under tension. Both the opposing muscle group (the muscles behind or in front) and the muscles to be stretched are relaxed. Then slowly and cautiously the body is moved to increase the tension of the muscle, or group of muscles, to be stretched. At this point the position is held or maintained to allow the muscles and tendons to lengthen.

This second part of an effective warm-up is extremely important: it helps to lengthen both the muscles and tendons, which in turn allow the joints a greater range of movement. This is very important in the prevention of muscle and tendon injuries.

The above two elements form the basis or foundation for a complete and effective warm-up. It is extremely important that these two elements be completed properly before moving on to the next two elements. The proper completion of elements one and two prepare the athlete for the more specific and vigorous activities necessary for elements three and four.

SPORTS INJURY PREVENTION

Recent studies have shown that static stretching may have an adverse affect on muscle contraction speed and therefore impair performance in athletes involved in sports requiring high levels of power and speed (Cramer et al, 2005). It is for this reason that static stretching is conducted early in the warm-up routine and is always followed by sport-specific drills and dynamic stretching.

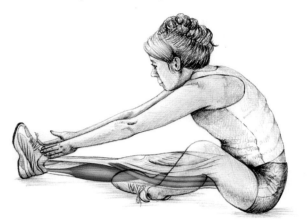

An example of static stretching.

3. Sport-specific warm-up

With the first two parts of the warm-up carried out thoroughly and correctly, it is now safe to move on to the third part of an effective warm-up. In this part, the athlete is specifically preparing their body for the demands of their particular sport. During this part of the warm-up, more vigorous activity should be employed. Activities should reflect the type of movements and actions that will be required during the sporting event.

4. Dynamic stretching

Finally, a correct warm-up should finish with a series of dynamic stretches. A note of caution: this form of stretching carries with it a high risk of injury if used incorrectly. Dynamic stretching is for muscular conditioning as well as flexibility and is really only suited for well-trained, highly conditioned athletes. Dynamic stretching should only be used after a high level of general flexibility has been established.

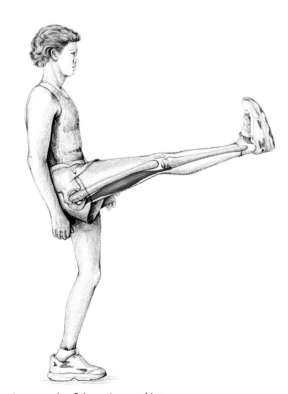

Dynamic stretching involves a controlled, soft bounce or swinging motion to move a particular body part to the limit of its range of movement. The force of the bounce or swing is gradually increased but should never become radical or uncontrolled.

During this last part of an effective warm-up it is also important to keep the dynamic stretches specific to the athlete's particular sport. This is the final part of the warm-up and should result in the athlete reaching a

An example of dynamic stretching.

physical and mental peak. At this point the athlete is most prepared for the rigours of their sport or activity.

The above information forms the basis of a complete and effective warm-up. However, the process described above is somewhat of an ideal or perfect warm-up. This is not always possible or convenient in the real world. In practice the individual athlete must be responsible for assessing their own goals and adjusting their warm-up accordingly.

For instance, the time committed to the warm-up should be relative to the level of involvement in the athlete's particular sport. For people only looking to increase their general level of health and fitness, a warm-up of 5–10 minutes would be enough. However, if involved in high-level competitive sport the athlete will need to dedicate adequate time and effort to a more extensive and complete warm-up.

COOL-DOWN

Many people dismiss the cool-down as a waste of time. In reality the cool-down is just as important as the warm-up, and if you are trying to stay injury free it is vital.

Although the warm-up and cool-down are equally important, they are important for different reasons. While the main purpose of warming-up is to prepare the body and mind for strenuous activity, cooling-down plays a very different role.

Why Cool-down?
The main aim of the cool-down is to promote recovery and return the body to a pre-exercise or pre-workout state. During a strenuous workout, the body goes through a number of stressful processes; muscle fibres, tendons and ligaments get damaged, and waste products build up. The cool-down, when performed properly, will assist the body in its repair process, and one area the cool-down will specifically help with is post-exercise muscle soreness. Another common term used for post-exercise muscle soreness is delayed-onset muscle soreness or DOMS.

This is the soreness that is usually experienced the day after a tough workout. Most people experience this after having a break from exercise or at the beginning of their sports season. An example would be running a 10km fun run or half marathon with very little preparation, and finding it difficult to walk down steps the next day because the quadriceps muscles are sore. This discomfort is post-exercise muscle soreness.

Post-exercise muscle soreness is caused by a number of factors. First, during exercise, tiny tears called microtears develop within the muscle fibres. These microtears cause swelling which in turn puts pressure on the nerve endings and results in pain.

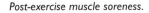

Post-exercise muscle soreness.

Second, when exercising, the heart pumps large amounts of blood to the working muscles. This blood carries the oxygen and nutrients that the working muscles need. When the blood reaches the muscles the oxygen and nutrients are used up and the force of the contracting (exercising) muscles pushes the blood back to the heart where it is re-oxygenated. However, when the exercise stops, so does the force that pushes the blood back to the heart. This blood, as well as waste products such as lactic acid, stays in the muscles, which in turn causes swelling and pain. This process is often referred to as blood pooling.

The cool-down helps keep the blood circulating, which in turn helps to prevent blood pooling and also removes waste products from the muscles. This circulating blood brings with it the oxygen and nutrients needed by the muscles, tendons and ligaments for repair.

The Key Parts of an Effective Cool-down

Now that the importance of the cool-down has been established, let us have a look at the structure of an effective cool-down. There are three key elements, or parts, which should be included to ensure an effective and complete cool-down. They are: gentle exercise, stretching and re-fuel.

All three elements are equally important and any one part should not be neglected or thought of as unnecessary. They work together to repair and replenish the body after exercise.

To follow are two examples of effective cool-downs. The first is an example of a typical cool-down that would be used by a professional athlete. The second is typical of someone who simply exercises for general health, fitness and fun.

Cool-down Routines for the Professional
- Start with 10–15 minutes of easy exercise. Be sure that the easy exercise resembles the type of exercise that was done during the workout. For example, if the workout involved a lot of running, cool-down with easy jogging or walking.
- Include some deep breathing as part of the easy exercise to help oxygenate the body.
- Follow with 20–30 minutes of stretching. Static stretching and proprioceptive neuromuscular facilitation (PNF) stretching are best for the cool-down.
- Re-fuel. Both fluid and food are important. Drink plenty of water, plus a good-quality sports drink. The best type of food to eat straight after a workout is that which is easily digestible. Fruit is a good example.

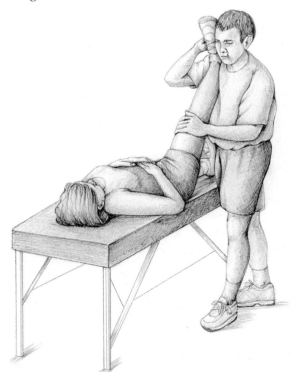

An example of PNF stretching.

Cool-down Routines for the Amateur
- Start with 3–5 minutes of easy exercise. Be sure that the easy exercise resembles the type of exercise that was done during the workout. For example, if the workout involved swimming or cycling, cool-down with a few easy laps of the pool or a slow ride around the block.
- Include some deep breathing as part of the easy exercise to help oxygenate the body.
- Follow with 5–10 minutes of stretching. Static stretching and PNF stretching are best for the cool-down.
- Re-fuel. Both fluid and food are important. Drink plenty of water, plus a good-quality sports drink. The best type of food to eat straight after a workout is that which is easily digestible. Fruit is a good example.

THE FITT PRINCIPLE

The FITT principle (or formula) is a great way of monitoring an exercise program. The acronym outlines the essential elements of an effective exercise program and the initials stand for:

F: Frequency   **I**: Intensity   **T**: Time   **T**: Type

Frequency
Frequency refers to the frequency of exercise undertaken or how the number of times the athlete exercises per week. Frequency is a key component of the FITT principle. Frequency needs to be adjusted to reflect: the athlete's current fitness level; the time the athlete realistically has available (considering other commitments like family and work); and the specific goals that the athlete has set for themself.

Intensity
Intensity refers to the intensity of exercise undertaken or how hard the athlete exercises. This is an extremely important aspect of the FITT principle and is probably the hardest factor to monitor. The best way to gauge the intensity of any exercise performed is to monitor heart rate.

There are a number of ways to monitor heart rate but the best way is to use an exercise heart rate monitor. These can be purchased at most sports stores and consist of an elastic belt that fits around the chest and a wrist watch that displays the exercise heart rate in beats per minute.

Time
Time refers to the time spent exercising or how long the athlete exercises for. The time dedicated to exercise usually depends on the type of exercise undertaken.

For example, at least 20–30 minutes of non-stop exercise is recommended to improve cardiovascular fitness. For weight loss, more time is required – at least 40 minutes of moderate weightbearing exercise. However, when talking about what exercise is required for muscular strength improvement, this is often measured as a number of sets and reps (repetitions). A typical recommendation would be three sets of eight reps.

Type
Type refers to the type of exercise undertaken or what kind of exercise the athlete does. Like time, the type of exercise chosen will have a big effect on the results achieved.

For example, if improving cardiovascular fitness is the goal, exercises like walking, jogging, swimming, bike riding, stair climbing, aerobics and rowing are very effective. For weight loss, any exercise that uses the majority of our large muscle groups will be effective. To improve muscular strength the best exercises include the use of free weights, machine weights and body weight exercises like push-ups, chin-ups and dips.

How Does All This Relate to Injury Prevention?

The two biggest mistakes people make when designing an exercise program are to train too hard and to not include enough variety.

The problem, most commonly, is that people tend to find an exercise they like and very rarely do anything other than that exercise. This can result in long-term, repetitive strain to the same muscle groups and neglect, or weakening, of other muscle groups. This will lead to an unbalanced muscular system, which is a sure-fire recipe for injury.

When using the FITT principle to design an exercise program, keep the following in mind:

Frequency

After exercise the body goes through a process of rebuilding and repair. It is during this process that the benefits of exercise are forthcoming.

However, if strenuous exercise is conducted on a daily basis (5–6 times a week) the body never has a chance to realize the benefits and gains from the exercise. In this case, what usually happens is that the athlete ends up getting tired or injured, or just quits.

To avoid this scenario, allow more rest and relaxation time, and cut down the frequency of strenuous exercise to only 3–4 times a week.

This may sound strange and a little hard to do at first, because most people have been conditioned into believing that they have to exercise every day, but after a while exercising like this becomes very enjoyable and something that can be looked forward to.

Exercising this way also dramatically reduces the likelihood of injury because the body has more time to repair and heal. Many elite level athletes have seen big improvements in performance when forced to take an extended break. Most never realize they are training too hard or too often.

Intensity and Time

The key here is variety. Do not get stuck in an exercise rut. Dedicate some of the workouts to long, easy sessions like long walks or light, repetitive weights. Other sessions can be made up of short, high-intensity exercises such as stair climbing or interval training.

Type

The type of exercise undertaken is also very important. Many people get into a routine of doing the same exercise over and over again. If lowering the risk of injury is the goal, do a variety of different exercises. This will benefit all the major muscle groups and will also help to make the athlete more versatile and well-rounded.

OVERTRAINING

There is a big difference between being just a little tired or on a down-cycle and being legitimately run down or overtrained. It is important to be able to tell the difference so as to remain injury free. Nothing will put a stop to improved sporting performance more quickly than not being able to recognize the signs of being legitimately run down and overtrained.

One of the biggest challenges to achieving fitness goals is consistency. If the athlete is repeatedly getting sick, run down and overtrained it becomes very difficult to stay injury free. The following information will help athletes keep the consistency of regular exercise, without overdoing it and becoming sick or injured.

Amateur and professional athletes alike are constantly battling with the problem of overtraining. Being able to juggle just the right amount of training with enough sleep and rest and the right nutrition is not an easy act to master. Throw in a career and a family and it becomes extremely difficult.

What is Overtraining?

Overtraining is the result of giving the body more work or stress than it can handle. Overtraining occurs when a person experiences stress and physical trauma from exercise faster than their body can repair the damage.

This does not happen overnight or as the result of one or two workouts. In fact, regular exercise is extremely beneficial to general health and fitness, but the athlete must always remember that it is exercise that breaks the body down, while it is rest and recovery that make the body strong and healthy. Improvements only occur during the times of rest.

Stress can come from a multitude of sources. It is not just physical stress that causes overtraining. Sure, excessive exercise coupled with inadequate rest will lead to overtraining, but do not forget to consider other stresses such as family or work commitments. Remember: stress is stress. Whether it is a physical, mental or emotional stress, it still has the same effect on the health and wellbeing of the body.

Reading the Signs

At this point in time there are no tests that can be performed to determine whether an athlete is overtrained or not. The athlete cannot go to a local doctor or even to a sports medicine laboratory and ask for a test for overtraining. However, while there are no tests for overtraining, there are a number of signs and symptoms that need to be watched out for. These signs and symptoms will act as a warning bell giving advance notice of possible dangers to come.

There are quite a number of signs and symptoms to be on the lookout for. To make them easier to recognize they are grouped below into either physical or psychological signs and symptoms.

Suffering from one or two of the following signs or symptoms does not automatically mean an athlete is suffering from overtraining. However, if a number (say five or six) are present, it may be time to take a closer look at the volume and intensity of the current workload.

Physical Signs and Symptoms

- Elevated resting pulse/heart rate
- Frequent minor infections
- Increased susceptibility to colds and influenza
- Increases in minor injuries
- Chronic muscle soreness or joint pain
- Exhaustion
- Lethargy
- Weight loss
- Appetite loss
- Insatiable thirst or dehydration

- Intolerance to exercise
- Decreased performance
- Delayed recovery from exercise

Psychological Signs and Symptoms

- Tired, drained or lacking energy
- Reduced ability to concentrate
- Apathy or lack of motivation
- Irritability
- Anxiety
- Depression
- Headaches
- Insomnia
- Inability to relax
- Twitchy, fidgety or jittery

As seen by the number of signs and symptoms, there is a lot to look out for. Generally the most common signs and symptoms of overtraining are a loss of motivation in all areas of life (work or career, health and fitness etc.) plus a feeling of exhaustion. If these two warning signs are present, plus a couple of the other listed signs and symptoms, then it may be time to take a short rest before things get out of hand.

The Answer to the Problem

Let us consider the following example. We feel run down and totally exhausted. We have no motivation to do anything. We cannot get rid of that niggling knee injury. We are irritable, depressed and have totally lost our appetite. Sounds like we are overtrained, but what do we do now?

As with most things, prevention is better than cure. To follow are a few measures that can be taken to prevent overtraining.

- Only make small and gradual increases to an exercise program over a period of time.
- Eat a well-balanced, nutritious diet.
- Be sure to get enough relaxation and sleep.
- Be prepared to modify the training routine to suit environmental conditions. For example, on a very hot day go to the pool instead of running on the track.
- Monitor other life stresses and make adjustments to suit.
- Avoid monotonous training by varying exercise routines as much as possible.
- Do not exercise during an illness.
- Be flexible and have some fun with the exercise undertaken.

While prevention should always be the aim, there will be times when overtraining will occur and the following information will help to get the overtrained athlete back on track.

The first priority is to take a rest; anywhere from 3–5 days should do the trick, depending on how severe the overtraining is. During this time the athlete needs to forget about exercise, and the body needs a rest too, so give it one – a physical rest, as well as a mental rest.

Try to get as much sleep and relaxation as possible. Go to bed early and catch a nap whenever possible. Increase the intake of highly nutritious foods and take an extra dose of vitamins and minerals.

After the initial 3–5 days rest the athlete can gradually get back into the normal exercise routine, but start off slowly. Most research states that it is fine to start off with the same intensity and time of exercise but cut back on the frequency. So if the athlete would normally exercise 3–4 times a week, cut that back to only twice a week for the next week or two. After that the athlete should be safe to resume the normal exercise regime.

Sometimes it is a good idea to have a rest, like the one outlined above, whether feeling run down or not. It will give both the mind and body a chance to fully recover from any problems that may be building up without the athlete even knowing it. It will also freshen up the mind, give a renewed motivation, and help the athlete look forward to exercise again. Do not underestimate the benefits of a good rest.

FITNESS AND SKILL DEVELOPMENT

An individual's physical fitness is made up of many components. The main ones are strength, power, speed, endurance, flexibility, balance, coordination, agility and skill. Although particular sports require different levels of each fitness component it is essential to plan a regular exercise or training program that covers all of the main components.

A common mistake made by athletes is to excessively focus on the components that are easily recognized within their particular sport and neglect the others. Although one component may be used more than another, it is important to see each component as only one spoke in the fitness wheel. An imbalance in one component may contribute to sports injury.

For example, football relies heavily on strength and power; however, the exclusion of skill drills and flexibility training may lead to serious injury and poor performance. Strength and flexibility are of prime concern to a gymnast but a sound training program would also improve power, speed and endurance.

The same is true for each individual. While some people seem to be naturally strong or flexible, it would be very unwise for such a person to completely ignore the other components of physical fitness. This is why athletes such as ironmen and triathletes are often referred to as being totally fit; their sports demand an even distribution of the components that make up physical fitness.

Defining the appropriate balance is the key to health and fitness success and staying injury free. This may require the assistance of a qualified professional trainer. To help with the implementation of an exercise or training program, four common training methods are discussed in detail below. They are strength training, circuit training, cross training and plyometric training.

Fitness
1: Strength Training
Strength training has been a part of sports conditioning for many years. It is touted for its effects on speed, strength, agility and muscle mass. Often overlooked though are its benefits for injury prevention.

What is Strength Training?

Strength training is moving the joints through a range of motion against resistance requiring the muscles to expend energy and contract forcefully to move the bones. Strength training can be done using various types of resistance and with or without equipment. Strength training is used to strengthen the muscles, tendons, bones and ligaments and to increase muscle mass.

Strength training should be implemented in the conditioning program of all sports, not just strength sports. The increase in speed, strength, agility and muscular endurance will benefit athletes of every sport.

Types of Strength Training

Strength training comes in a variety of formats. The formats are described by the type of resistance and equipment used.

Machine Weights

Machine strength training includes resistance exercises done using any of the various machines designed to produce resistance. These include machines with weight stacks, hydraulics, resistance rods or bands, and even the use of theraband or resistance tubing.

The resistance, or weight, may be changed to increase the intensity of the exercise. The range of motion and position of movement is controlled by the machine. The resistance may be constant throughout the movement or may change due to the set-up of the pulley or hydraulic systems. Machines often add a degree of safety but neglect the stabilizer, or helper, muscles in a movement.

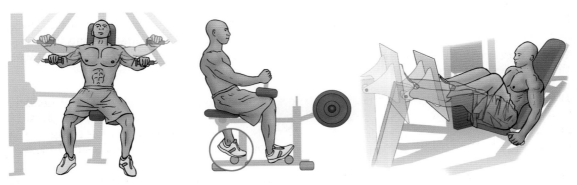

Examples of machine weights.

Free Weights

Free weight strength training involves using weights that are not fixed in a movement pattern by a machine. These include barbells and dumbbells. Also included in this group are kettlebells, medicine balls, ankle and wrist weights and weightlifting chains.

The weight used, as with the machines, may be changed to increase the resistance of an exercise. The resistance at different points along the range of motion transfers to different muscles and due to angles may lessen at times. At the limit of a joint's range of motion the weight is transferred to the joint as the muscles simply stabilize the joint.

The range of motion and path of movement is not limited so the stabilizing muscles must work to keep the joints in line during the movement. Due to the fact that the movement is not fixed, poor form can become an issue.

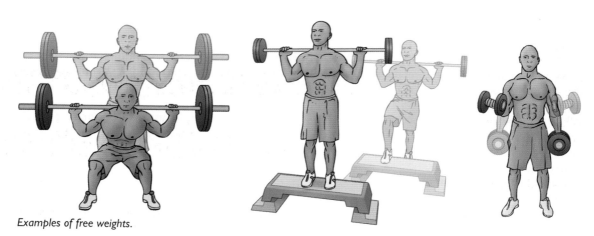

Examples of free weights.

Own Bodyweight Exercises

Bodyweight exercises utilize the athlete's bodyweight as resistance during the exercise. As with free weights, the range and path of motion is not fixed by a machine. Exercises such as plyometric jumping, push-ups, pull-ups, abdominal exercises, even sprinting and jumping rope, fall into this category.

The weight used in these exercises is constant and only changes when the athlete's body changes. The changes in resistance during the movement are similar to those of free weight exercises.

The range of motion and path of movement does not follow a fixed path so stabilizing muscles come into play. Form is again an issue with these exercises. The inability to change the weight used does limit the effectiveness for some athletes. Larger athletes will be limited in the exercises they can perform and the number of repetitions. Smaller athletes will quickly go beyond the desired repetition range for strength building.

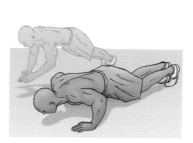
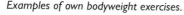
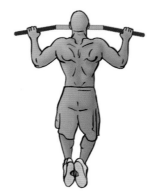
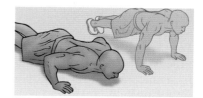

Examples of own bodyweight exercises.

How Does Strength Training Prevent Injury?

Strength training in athletics is common practice today. The benefits are obvious and the immediate crossover of those benefits to the playing field makes it ideal for off-season conditioning. Injury prevention is one benefit that is often overlooked. Strength training is a very effective tool for injury prevention for a variety of reasons.

Strength training improves the strength of the muscles, tendons and even the ligaments and bones. The stronger muscles and tendons help to hold the body in proper alignment and protect the bones and joints when moving or under impact. The bones become stronger due to the load placed on them during training, and the ligaments become more flexible and better at absorbing the shock applied to them during dynamic movements.

When an area of the body is used less during an activity it may become weaker than the other areas. This can become a problem when that area (whether a muscle, ligament, joint or specific bone) is called into play suddenly. If the area cannot handle the sudden stress placed on it an injury may occur. Strength training, using a balanced programme, will eliminate these weak areas and balance the body for the activities it is called on to do.

Muscle imbalances are one of the most common causes of injuries in athletics. When one muscle, or muscle group, becomes stronger than its opposing group, the weaker muscles become fatigued quicker and more susceptible to injury. A forceful contraction near maximal output from the stronger muscle can also cause damage to the weaker opposing muscle due to its inability to counter the force.

Muscle imbalances also affect the joints and bones due to abnormal pull causing the joint to move in an unnatural pattern. The stronger muscles will cause the joint to pull in that direction, causing a stretching of the opposing ligaments and a tightening of the supporting ones. This can lead to chronic pain and an unnatural wearing of the bones. A balanced strength training program will help to counter these effects by strengthening the weaker muscles to balance them with their counterparts.

Precautions for Strength Training

Strength training is a great tool for injury prevention. Becoming injured during strength training obviously defeats this purpose. To avoid injury it is essential that proper form be used in all exercises. Keeping the body in proper alignment while exercising will minimize the chances of injury. Starting with light weights or resistance and developing proper form before increasing the resistance is important. When increasing the resistance it is important to do so in small increments and only when the desired number of repetitions can be performed in correct form.

Rest plays a crucial role in the efficiency and safety of a training program. Remember: muscles repair and become stronger during rest, not during the workout. Performing strength training exercises for the same muscle groups without adequate rest between training sessions can lead to overtraining. Overtraining will result in the muscles being unable to repair properly and not being ready for additional work. This can lead to acute or chronic injuries.

Fitness
2: Circuit Training

Circuit training routines are a favorite training session for many coaches and athletes. Circuit training can be used as part of injury rehabilitation programs, for conditioning elite level athletes, or to help with weight loss. Circuits can be used for just about everything.

Circuit training consists of a consecutive series of timed exercises performed one after the other with varying amounts of rest between each exercise.

For example, a simple circuit training routine might consist of push-ups, sit-ups, squats, chin-ups and lunges. The routine might be structured as follows, and could be continually repeated as many times as is necessary.

- Do as many push-ups as possible in 30 seconds, then rest for 30 seconds.
- Do as many squats as possible in 30 seconds, then rest for 30 seconds.
- Do as many sit-ups as possible in 30 seconds, then rest for 30 seconds.
- Do as many lunges as possible in 30 seconds, then rest for 30 seconds.
- Do as many chin-ups as possible in 30 seconds, then rest for 30 seconds.

What Makes Circuit Training So Good?
The quick pace and constant changing nature of circuit training places a unique type of stress on the body, which differs from normal exercise activities such as weight training and aerobic exercise.

The demands of circuit training prepare the body in a very even, all-round manner. Circuit training is an exceptional form of exercise to aid in the prevention of injury and is one of the best ways to condition the entire body and mind.

There are many other reasons why circuit training is a fantastic form of exercise and what most of these reasons come down to is flexibility. In other words, circuit training is totally adaptable to the specific requirements of the individual.

- Circuit training can be totally personalized. Whether a beginner or an elite athlete, circuit training routines can be modified to give the best possible results.
- A circuit training routine can be modified to give the athlete exactly what they want. Whether for an all-over body workout, or just working on a specific body area or aspect of the chosen sport, this can all be accommodated.
- It is easy to change the focus of the circuit training routine to emphasize strength, endurance, agility, speed, skill development, weight loss or any other aspect of fitness that is important to the individual.
- Circuit training is time efficient. With no wasted time in between sets, it gives maximum results in minimum time.
- Circuit training can be done just about anywhere. Circuit training is a favorite form of exercise for British Royal Marines commandos because they spend a lot of time on large ships. The confined space means that circuit training is sometimes the only form of exercise available to them.
- No expensive equipment is needed – not even a gym membership. It is just as easy to put together a great circuit training routine at home or in a park. By using some imagination it is easy to devise all sorts of exercises using things like chairs and tables, and even children's outdoor play equipment like swings and monkey bars.
- Another reason why circuit training is so popular is that it is great fun to do in pairs or groups. Half the group performs the exercises while the other half rests and motivates the exercising members of the group.

Types of Circuit Training

As mentioned before, circuit training can be totally customized, which means there are an unlimited number of ways to structure a circuit training routine. Here are a few examples of the different types available:

Timed Circuit
This type of circuit involves working to a set time period for both rest and exercise intervals. For example, a typical timed circuit might involve 30 seconds of exercise and 30 seconds of rest in between each exercise.

Competition Circuit

This is similar to a timed circuit but each individual pushes themself to see how many repetitions can be done in a set time period. (For example, complete 12 push-ups in 30 seconds.) The idea is to keep the time period the same but try to increase the number of repetitions achieved within it.

Repetition Circuit

This type of circuit is great when working with large groups of people who have different levels of fitness and ability. The idea is that the fittest group might do 20 repetitions of each exercise; the intermediate group might only do 15 repetitions; while the beginners might only do 10 repetitions of each exercise.

Sport-specific or Running Circuit

This type of circuit is best done outside or in a large, open area with exercises that are specific to the participants' sport, or emphasize an aspect of the sport that needs improvement. Then instead of simply resting between exercises run easy for 200–400 metres.

Some Important Precautions

Circuit training is a fantastic form of exercise. However, the most common problem is that people tend to get over excited, because of the timed nature of the exercises, and push themselves harder than they normally would. This tends to result in sore muscles and joints and an increased likelihood of injury. Below are two precautions to take into consideration:

Level of Fitness

If the athlete has never done any sort of circuit training before, even if they are considered quite fit, start off slowly. The nature of circuit training is quite different to any other form of exercise. It places different demands on the body and mind and, if the athlete is not used to it, it will take a few sessions for the body to adapt to this new form of training.

Warm-up and Cool-down

Do not ever start a circuit training routine without a thorough warm-up that includes stretching. As mentioned previously, circuit training is very different from other forms of exercise. The body must be prepared for circuit training before starting a session.

Fitness
3: Cross Training

Cross training, although it has been used for years, is relatively new as a training concept. Athletes have been forced to use exercises outside their sport for conditioning for many reasons, including: weather, seasonal change, facility and equipment availability, and injuries. These athletes were cross training whether they knew it or not. The benefits of cross training are beginning to get more press and one of those is injury prevention.

What Is Cross Training?

Cross training is the use of various activities to achieve overall conditioning. Cross training uses activities outside the normal drills and exercises commonly associated with a sport. The exercises provide a break from the normal impact of training in a particular sport, thereby giving the muscles, tendons, bones, joints and ligaments a brief break. These exercises target the muscles from a different angle or resistance and work to balance an athlete. Cross training is an effective way of resting the body from the usual sport-specific activities while maintaining conditioning.

Any exercise or activity can be used for cross training if it is not a skill associated with that particular sport. Weight training is a commonly used cross training tool. Swimming, cycling, running and even skiing are activities used for cross training. Plyometrics are becoming popular again as cross training tools.

Critics of Cross Training

Cross training does help achieve balance in the muscles due to working them from various angles and in different positions. Cross training does not, however, develop skills specific to the sport or sport-specific conditioning. A football player who jogs three to five miles all summer and lifts weights will still not be in football shape when the preseason starts. Cross training cannot be used as the sole conditioning tool. Sport-specific conditioning and skill training is still required.

High-impact sports such as basketball, gymnastics, football and running cause a lot of jarring to the skeletal system. Cross training can help limit the jarring but some sport-specific impact is necessary to condition athletes for their activity. A runner who runs in water as their only conditioning routine may develop shin splints and other injuries when they are required to run on hard surfaces for races or training. Their body is not conditioned to the forces it is subjected to and will react accordingly.

Jumping into an intense cross training schedule without progressing into it properly can also lead to problems. It is important to progressively increase the intensity, duration and frequency in small increments.

Cross Training Examples

Cross training can take many forms. The key to a successful cross training program is that it must address the same energy systems used in the sport and must allow a break from sport-specific activities. Training the same major muscle groups in a different way keeps the athlete conditioned but helps prevent overuse injuries

- A cyclist may use swimming to build upper body strength and to maintain cardiovascular endurance. They may use cross-country skiing to maintain leg strength and endurance when snow and ice eliminate biking time.
- Swimmers may use free weight training to develop and maintain strength levels. They may incorporate rock climbing to keep upper body strength and endurance up.
- Runners may use mountain biking to target the legs from a slightly different approach. They can use deep water running to lessen the impact while still maintaining a conditioning schedule.
- A shot putter may use Olympic weightlifting exercises to build overall explosiveness. They may use plyometrics and sprinting to develop explosiveness in the hips and legs.

How Does Cross Training Prevent Injury?

Cross training is an important tool in the injury prevention program of athletes. Cross training allows coaches and athletes the opportunity to train hard all year round without running the risk of overtraining or overuse injuries. The simple process of changing the type of training changes the stress on the body.

Cross training gives the muscles used in the primary sport a break from the normal stresses put on them each day. The muscles may still be worked, even intensely, but without the normal impact or from a different angle. This allows the muscles to recover from the wear and tear that builds up over a season. This active rest is a much better recovery tool than total rest and forces the body to adapt to different stimuli.

Cross training also helps to reduce or reverse muscle imbalances in the body. A pitcher in baseball may develop an imbalance laterally between the two sides of the body as well as in the shoulder girdle of the throwing arm. Thousands of pitches over a season will cause the muscles directly involved in throwing to become stronger while supporting muscles and those unaffected by throwing will become weaker without training. Cross training can help balance the strength in the muscles on both sides as well as the stabilizing muscles. This balancing of strength and flexibility helps to prevent one muscle group, due to a strength imbalance, from pulling the body out of natural alignment. It also prevents muscle pulls and tears caused by one muscle exerting more force than the opposing group can counter.

Precautions for Cross Training
Whenever starting a new activity it is important to get instruction in the proper techniques and safety measures. For example, ocean kayaking can be a great cross training activity for tennis players to develop and maintain upper body endurance but without instruction on proper techniques it can be dangerous.

Equipment used for cross training activities should be fitted properly and designed for the activity. Unsafe or ill-fitted equipment can lead to injury.

Cross training is a great way to avoid overuse injuries and overtraining. Unfortunately, these same pitfalls can be an issue in a cross training programme. Varying workouts, adequate rest between workouts, use of proper form and gradual increasing resistance are important in any programme. Many athletes simply add cross training to their current programme rather than substituting. This leads to overtraining and the opposite of the injury prevention goal.

Fitness
Part 4: Plyometric Training
The previous three sections looked at three very good training techniques to help develop and condition athletic ability, which in turn will help to prevent sports injury. This section will build on the last three techniques by discussing a slightly more advanced form of athletic conditioning called plyometrics.

What Are Plyometric Exercises?
In the simplest of terms, plyometrics are exercises that involve a jumping movement. For example, side-to-side jumping, bounding, jumping rope, punchbag push, hopping, lunges, trunk curl and throw, jump squats, and clap push-ups are all examples of plyometric exercises.

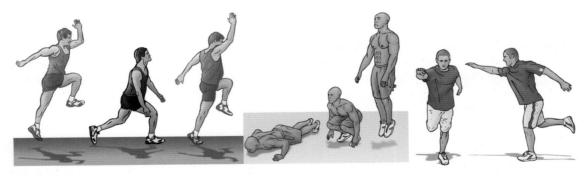

Examples of plyometric training.

However, for a more detailed definition some background information about muscle contractions is needed. Muscles contract in one of three ways:

1. Eccentric Muscle Contraction

An eccentric muscle contraction occurs when the muscle contracts and lengthens at the same time. An example of an eccentric muscle contraction is lowering an object held in the hand down to your side. The biceps brachii (upper arm) muscle contracts eccentrically to enable controlled lowering of the arm.

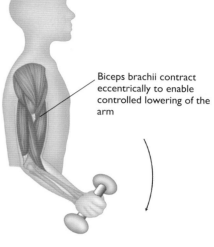

Biceps brachii contract eccentrically to enable controlled lowering of the arm

2. Concentric Muscle Contraction

A concentric muscle contraction occurs when the muscle contracts and shortens at the same time. An example of a concentric muscle contraction is lifting the body up into a chin-up position. The biceps brachii muscle contracts and shortens as the body is raised up to the chin-up bar.

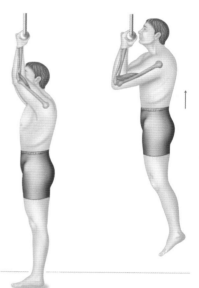

3. Isometric Muscle Contraction

An isometric muscle contraction occurs when the muscle contracts but does not change in length. An example of an isometric muscle contraction is holding a heavy object in the hand with the elbow held stationary and bent at 90 degrees. The biceps brachii muscle contracts but does not change in length because the body is not moving up or down.

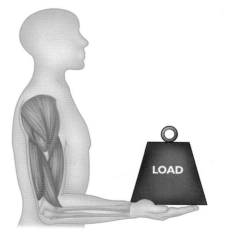

LOAD

Getting back to the formal definition, a plyometric exercise is an exercise in which an eccentric muscle contraction is quickly followed by a concentric muscle contraction. In other words, when a muscle is rapidly contracted and lengthened, then immediately followed with a further contraction and shortening, this is a plyometric exercise. This process of contract-lengthen, contract-shorten is often referred to as the stretch-shortening cycle.

Here is another example of a plyometric exercise. Consider the simple act of jumping off a step, landing on the ground with both feet and then jumping forward, all in one swift movement.

When jumping off the step and landing on the ground, the muscles in the legs contract eccentrically to slow the body down. When jumping forward the muscles contract concentrically to spring off the ground. This is a classic example of a plyometric exercise.

Why Are Plyometric Exercises Important for Injury Prevention?

Athletes often use plyometrics to develop power for their chosen sport, and a lot has been written about how to accomplish this. However, few people realize how important plyometrics can be in aiding injury prevention.

Essentially, plyometric exercises force the muscle to contract rapidly from a full stretch position. This is the position in which muscles tend to be at their weakest. By conditioning the muscle at its weakest point (full stretch) it is better prepared to handle this type of stress in a real or game environment.

Why Are Plyometric Exercises Important for Injury Rehabilitation?

Most injury rehabilitation programs fail to realize that an eccentric muscle contraction can be up to three times more forceful than a concentric muscle contraction. This is why plyometric exercises are important in the final stage of rehabilitation, to condition the muscles to handle the added strain of eccentric contractions.

Neglecting this final stage of the rehabilitation process can often lead to re-injury, because the muscles have not been conditioned to cope with the added force of eccentric muscle contractions.

Caution, Caution, Caution!
Plyometrics are NOT for everyone. Plyometric exercises are not for the amateur and they are not for the weekend warrior. They are an advanced form of athletic conditioning and can place a massive strain on unconditioned muscles, joints and bones.

Plyometric exercises should only be used by well-conditioned athletes and preferably under the supervision of a professional sports coach. When adding plyometric exercises to a regular training routine, please take careful note of the following precautions.

- Children or teenagers who are still growing should not use intense, repetitive plyometric exercises.
- A solid base of muscular strength and endurance should be developed before starting a plyometrics program. In fact Better-Body.com recommends: "It is a good rule of thumb that before we start using any plyometric exercises we should be able to squat at least 1.5 times our own body weight, and then focus on developing core strength."
- A thorough warm-up is essential to ensure the athlete is ready for the intensity of plyometric exercises.
- Do not perform plyometric exercises on concrete, asphalt or other hard surfaces. Grass is one of the best surfaces for plyometric exercises.

- Technique is important. As soon as form deteriorates or the athlete feels tired, back off.
- Do not overdo it. Plyometrics are very intense. Allow plenty of rest between sessions, and do not perform plyometric exercises two days in a row.

STRETCHING AND FLEXIBILITY

1: How Does Stretching Prevent Sports Injury?

Stretching is a simple and effective activity that helps to enhance athletic performance, decrease the likelihood of injury and minimize muscle soreness. But how specifically does stretching prevent sports injury?

Improved Range of Movement

By placing particular parts of the body in certain positions, we are able to increase the length of our muscles. As a result of this, a reduction in general muscle tension is achieved and our normal range of movement is increased.

By increasing our range of movement we are increasing the distance our limbs can move before damage occurs to the muscles and tendons. For example, the muscles and tendons in the back of the leg are put under great strain when kicking a football. Therefore, the more flexible and pliable those muscles are, the further the leg can travel forward before a strain or injury occurs to them.

The benefits of an extended range of movement include: increased comfort; a greater ability to move freely; and a lessening of our susceptibility to muscle and tendon strain injuries.

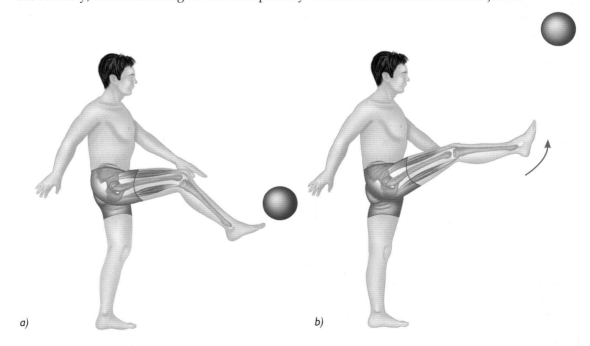

a)   *b)*

Improved range of movement when kicking a football; a) limited range of movement, b) improved range of movement after conditioning.

Reduced Post-exercise Muscle Soreness

We have all experienced what happens when we go for a run or to the gym for the first time in a few months. The following day our muscles are tight, sore and stiff, and it is usually hard to even walk down a flight of stairs. The soreness that usually accompanies strenuous physical activity is often referred to as post-exercise muscle soreness. This soreness is the result of microtears, (minute tears within the muscle fibres), blood pooling and accumulated waste products such as lactic acid. Stretching, as part of an effective cool-down, helps to alleviate this soreness by lengthening the individual muscle fibres, increasing blood circulation and removing waste products.

Reduced Fatigue

Fatigue is a major problem for everyone, especially those who exercise. It results in a decrease in both physical and mental performance. Increased flexibility through stretching can help prevent the effects of fatigue by taking pressure off the working muscle (the agonist). For every muscle in the body there is an opposite or opposing muscle, (the antagonist). If the opposing muscles are more flexible, the working muscles do not have to exert as much force against the opposing muscles. Therefore each movement of the working muscles actually takes less effort.

Added Benefits

Along with the benefits listed above, a regular stretching program will also help to improve posture, develop body awareness, improve coordination, promote circulation, increase energy and improve relaxation and stress relief.

2: The Rules for Safe Stretching

As with most activities there are rules and guidelines to ensure that they are safe. Stretching is no exception. Stretching can be extremely dangerous and harmful if done incorrectly. It is vitally important that the following rules be adhered to, both for safety and for maximizing the potential benefits of stretching.

There is often confusion and concerns about which stretches are good and which stretches are bad. In most cases someone has told the enquirer that they should not do this stretch or that stretch, or that this is a good stretch and this is a bad stretch.

Are there only good stretches and bad stretches? Is there no middle ground? And if there are only good and bad stretches, how do we decide which ones are good and which ones are bad? Let us put an end to the confusion once and for all...

There is no such thing as a good or bad stretch!

Just as there are no good or bad exercises, there are no good or bad stretches – only what is appropriate for the specific requirements of the individual. So a stretch that is perfectly good for one person may not be right for someone else.

Let me use an example: a person with a shoulder injury would not be expected to do push-ups or freestyle swimming, but that does not mean that these are bad exercises. Now, consider the same scenario from a stretching point of view. That same person should avoid shoulder stretches, but that does not mean that all shoulder stretches are bad.

The stretch itself is neither good nor bad. It is the way the stretch is performed and by whom that makes stretching either effective and safe or ineffective and harmful. To place a particular stretch into a category of good or bad is unwise and potentially dangerous. To label a stretch as good gives people the impression that they can do that stretch whenever and however they want and it will not cause them any problems.

The specific requirements of the individual are what is important!

Remember, stretches are neither good nor bad. However, when choosing a stretch there are a number of precautions and checks we need to perform before giving that stretch the go-ahead.

1. First, make a general review of the individual. Are they healthy and physically active, or have they been leading a sedentary lifestyle for the past five years? Are they a professional athlete? Are they recovering from a serious injury? Do they have aches, pains or muscle and joint stiffness in any area of their body?

2. Second, make a specific review of the area or muscle group to be stretched. Are the muscles healthy? Is there any damage to the joints, ligaments or tendons? Has the area been injured recently or is it still recovering from an injury?

If the muscle group being stretched is not 100 per cent healthy, avoid stretching this area altogether. Work on recovery and rehabilitation before moving on to specific stretching exercises. If however, the individual is healthy and the area to be stretched is free from injury, then apply the following to all stretches.

Warm-up Prior to Stretching

This first rule is often overlooked and can lead to serious injury if not performed effectively. Trying to stretch muscles that have not been warmed is like trying to stretch old, dry rubber bands: they may snap.

Warming-up prior to stretching does a number of beneficial things but primarily its purpose is to prepare the body and mind for more strenuous activity. One of the ways it achieves this is by helping to increase the body's core temperature while also increasing the body's muscle temperature. By increasing muscle temperature we are helping to make the muscles loose and supple. This is essential to ensure the maximum benefit is gained from stretching.

The correct warm-up also has the effect of increasing both heart rate and respiratory rate. This increases blood flow, which in turn increases the delivery of oxygen and nutrients to the working muscles. All this helps to prepare the muscles for stretching.

A correct warm-up should consist of light physical activity. The fitness level of the participating athlete should govern both the intensity and duration of the warm-up, although a correct warm-up for most people should take about ten minutes and result in a light sweat.

Stretch Before and After Exercise

The question often arises: "Should I stretch before or after exercise?" This is not an either/or situation as both are essential. It is no good stretching after exercise and counting that as the pre-exercise stretch for next time. Stretching after exercise has a totally different purpose to stretching before exercise. The two are not the same.

The purpose of stretching before exercise is to help prevent injury. Stretching does this by lengthening the muscles and tendons, which in turn increases our range of movement. This ensures that we are able to move freely without restriction or injury occurring.

However, stretching after exercise has a very different role. Its purpose is primarily to aid in the repair and recovery of the muscles and tendons. By lengthening the muscles and tendons, stretching helps to prevent tight muscles and delayed muscle soreness that usually accompanies strenuous exercise.

After exercise our stretching should be done as part of a cool-down. The cool-down will vary depending on the duration and intensity of exercise undertaken, but will usually consist of 5–10 minutes of very light physical activity and be followed by 5–10 minutes of static stretching exercises.

An effective cool-down involving light physical activity and stretching will help to rid waste products from the muscles, prevent blood pooling and promote the delivery of oxygen and nutrients to the muscles. All this assists in returning the body to a pre-exercise level, thus aiding the recovery process.

Stretch All Major Muscles and Their Opposing Muscle Groups
When stretching, it is vitally important that we pay attention to all the major muscle groups in the body. Just because a particular sport may place a lot of emphasis on the legs, for example, does not mean that one can neglect the muscles of the upper body in a stretching routine.

All the muscles play an important part in any physical activity, not just a select few. Muscles in the upper body, for example, are extremely important in any running sport. They play a vital role in the stability and balance of the body during the running motion. Therefore it is important to keep them both flexible and supple.

Every muscle in the body has an opposing muscle that acts against it. For example, the muscles in the front of the thigh (the quadriceps) are opposed by the muscles in the back of the thigh (the hamstrings). These two groups of muscles provide a resistance to each other to balance the body. If one of these groups of muscles becomes stronger or more flexible than the other group, it is likely to lead to imbalances that can result in injury or postural problems.

For example, hamstring tears are a common injury in most running sports. They are often caused by strong quadriceps and weak, inflexible hamstrings. This imbalance puts a great deal of pressure on the hamstrings and can result in a muscle tear or strain.

Stretch Gently and Slowly
Stretching gently and slowly helps to relax our muscles, which in turn makes stretching more pleasurable and beneficial. This will also help to avoid muscle tears and strains that can be caused by rapid, jerky movements.

Stretch ONLY to the Point of Tension
Stretching is NOT an activity that is meant to be painful; it should be pleasurable, relaxing and very beneficial. Many people believe that to get the most from their stretching they need to be in constant pain. This is one of the greatest mistakes we can make when stretching. Let me explain why.

When the muscles are stretched to the point of pain, the body employs a defense mechanism called the stretch reflex. This is the body's safety measure to prevent serious damage occurring to the muscles, tendons and joints. The stretch reflex protects the muscles and tendons by contracting them, thereby preventing them from being stretched.

So to avoid the stretch reflex, avoid pain. Never push the stretch beyond what is comfortable. Only stretch to the point where tension can be felt in the muscles. This way, injury will be avoided and the maximum benefits from stretching will be achieved.

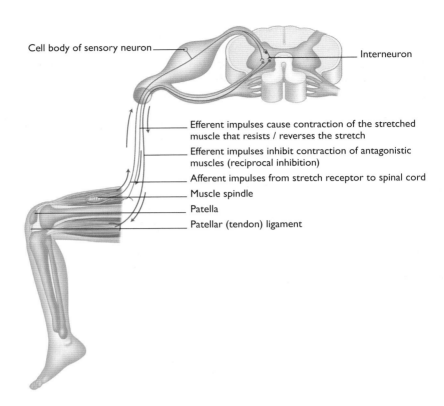

Cell body of sensory neuron

Interneuron

Efferent impulses cause contraction of the stretched muscle that resists / reverses the stretch

Efferent impulses inhibit contraction of antagonistic muscles (reciprocal inhibition)

Afferent impulses from stretch receptor to spinal cord

Muscle spindle

Patella

Patellar (tendon) ligament

The stretch reflex arc.

Breathe Slowly and Easily While Stretching

Many people unconsciously hold their breath while stretching. This causes tension in our muscles, which in turn makes it very difficult to stretch. To avoid this, remember to breathe slowly and deeply during all stretching exercises. This helps to relax our muscles, promotes blood flow and increases the delivery of oxygen and nutrients to our muscles.

An Example

By taking a look at one of the most controversial stretches ever performed, we can see how the above rules are applied. The stretch pictured opposite causes many a person to go into complete meltdown. It has a reputation as a dangerous, bad stretch that should be avoided at all cost. So why is it that at every Olympic Games, Commonwealth Games and World Championships, sprinters can be seen doing this stretch before their events? Let us apply the above checks to find out.

First, consider the person performing the stretch. Are they healthy, fit and physically active? If not, this is not a stretch they should be doing. Are they elderly, overweight or unfit? Are they young and still growing? Do they lead a sedentary lifestyle? If so, they should avoid this stretch! This first consideration alone would prohibit 50 per cent of the population from doing this stretch.

Second, review the area to be stretched. This stretch obviously puts a large strain on the muscles of the hamstrings and lower back. So if our hamstrings or lower back are not 100 per cent healthy, do not perform this stretch.

This second consideration would probably rule out another 25 per cent, which means this stretch is only suitable for about 25 per cent of the population: in other words the well-trained, physically fit, injury-free athlete.

Apply the six precautions above and the well-trained, physically fit, injury-free athlete can perform this stretch safely and effectively.

Remember, the stretch itself is neither good nor bad. It is the way the stretch is performed and by whom it is being performed that makes stretching either effective and safe or ineffective and harmful.

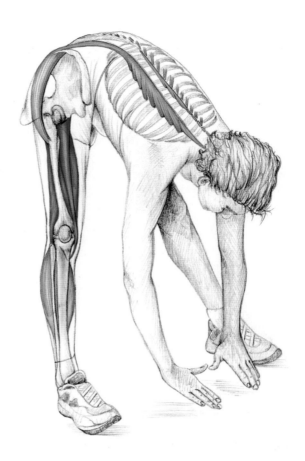

3: How to Stretch Properly

When to Stretch

Stretching is as important as the rest of an exercise programme. For the athlete involved in any competitive type of sport or exercise it is crucial to make time for specific stretching workouts. Set time aside to work on particular areas that are tight or stiff. The more involved and committed you are to your exercise and fitness, the more time and effort you will need to commit to stretching.

As discussed earlier it is important to stretch both before and after exercise. But when else should you stretch and what type of stretching is best for a particular purpose?

Choosing the right type of stretching for the right purpose will make a big difference to the effectiveness of your flexibility program. To follow are some suggestions for when to use the different types of stretches.

For warming-up dynamic stretching is the most effective, while for cooling-down static, passive and PNF stretching is best. For improving range of movement try PNF and active isolated stretching, and for rehabilitation a combination of PNF, isometric and active stretching will give the best results.

So when else should we stretch? Stretch periodically throughout the entire day. It is a great way to keep loose and to help ease the stress of everyday life. One of the most productive ways to utilize our time is to stretch while we are watching television. Start with five minutes of marching or jogging on the spot then take a seat on the floor in front of the television and start stretching.

Hold, Count, Repeat

For how long should I hold each stretch? How often should I stretch? For how long should I stretch?
These are the most commonly asked questions about stretching. Although there are conflicting responses to these questions, the answers given here are based on my study of research literature and personal experience and, I believe, reflect what is currently the most correct and beneficial information.

The question that causes the most disagreement is: *"For how long should I hold each stretch?"* Some sources state that as little as 10 seconds is enough. This is a bare minimum. Ten seconds is only just enough time for the muscles to relax and start to lengthen. For any real benefit to flexibility each stretch should be held for at least 20–30 seconds.

The time an individual commits to stretching will be relative to their level of involvement in a particular sport. For people looking to increase their general level of health and fitness a minimum of about 20 seconds will be enough. However, an athlete involved in high-level competitive sport will need to hold each stretch for at least 30 seconds and start to extend that to 60 seconds and beyond.

"How often should I stretch?"
How often an individual commits to stretching each muscle group will also be relative to their level of involvement in a particular sport. For example, the beginner should stretch each muscle group 2–3 times. However, the athlete participating at an advanced level in their sport should stretch each muscle group 3–5 times.

"For how long should I stretch?"
The same principle applies. For the beginner, about 5–10 minutes is enough, and for the professional athlete anything up to two hours. The individual participating somewhere between the beginner and the professional should adjust the time they spend stretching accordingly.

Please do not be impatient with stretching. Nobody can get fit in a couple of weeks so do not expect miracles from a stretching routine. Some muscle groups may need a minimum of three months of intense stretching to see any real improvement. Stick with it; it is well worth the effort.

Sequence

When starting a stretching program it is a good idea to start with general stretches for the entire body instead of just a select few. The idea of this is to reduce overall muscle tension and to increase the mobility of the joints and limbs.

The next step should be to increase overall flexibility by starting to extend the muscles and tendons beyond their normal range of movement. Following this, work on specific areas that are tight or important for a particular sport. Remember, all this takes time. This sequence of stretches may take up to three months to yield real improvement, especially for individuals with no background in agility-based activities or who are heavily muscled.

No data exists on what order stretches should be completed in. However, it is recommended to start with sitting stretches, because there is less chance of injury while sitting, before moving on to standing stretches. To make it easier you may want to start with the ankles and move up to the neck or vice versa. It really does not matter as long as all the major muscle groups and their opposing muscles are covered.

Once you have advanced beyond improving overall flexibility and are working on improving the range of movement of specific muscles, or muscle groups, it is important to isolate those muscles during stretching routines. To do this, concentrate on only one muscle group at a time. For example, instead of trying to stretch both hamstrings at the same time, concentrate on only one at a time. Stretching this way will help to reduce the resistance from other supporting muscle groups.

Posture

Posture or alignment while stretching is one of the most neglected aspects of flexibility training. It is important to be aware of how crucial it can be to the overall benefits of stretching. Bad posture and incorrect technique can cause imbalances in the muscles which can lead to injury; proper posture will ensure that the targeted muscle group receives the best possible stretch.

Major muscle groups are made up of a number of different muscles working together. If posture is sloppy or incorrect, stretching exercises can put more strain on one particular muscle in that muscle group, thus causing an imbalance that could lead to injury.

For example, when stretching the hamstrings (the muscles at the back of the legs) it is imperative to keep both feet pointing up. If the feet fall to one side this will put undue stress on one particular part of the hamstrings, which could result in a muscle imbalance.

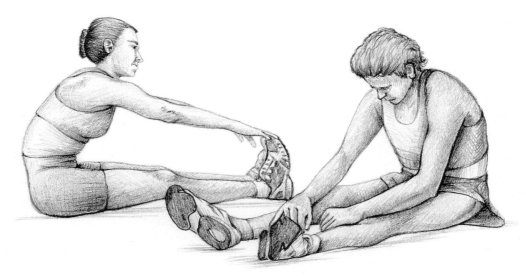

The difference between good and bad posture. Note the athlete on the left, feet upright and back relatively straight. The athlete on the right is at greater risk of causing a muscular imbalance that could lead to injury.

FACILITIES, RULES AND PROTECTIVE DEVICES

A number of less obvious prevention techniques are often overlooked but are equally important in helping to prevent sports injury.

Playing Areas and Facilities

These areas, designed specifically for sport and athletic activity, are often a source of unnecessary sports injuries. Broken, faulty or poorly designed equipment can lead to injury, and playing surfaces that are damaged or poorly maintained put athletes at unnecessary risk.

Before participation, ensure that playing areas are free from obstruction and in good condition. Spectators should also be made aware of the importance of staying well back from playing areas.

Rules

Sporting rules are specifically designed for the protection of players and ensure a safe playing area both for participants and spectators. It is the responsibility of coaching staff, players and referees to fully understand and abide by all the rules of their particular sport.

Emphasis should also be placed on good sportsmanship, fair play and the discouragement of dangerous or violent behavior.

Protective Devices

Protective devices are designed to aid performance and reduce injuries, with all sports participation benefiting from the use of protective devices. Even the sport of running is greatly enhanced with good supportive footwear and swimmers benefit from protective eye goggles.

Other important protective devices include: mouth guards; individual player pads; helmets; shin guards; eye protection; wetsuits; goalpost pads; and matting for sports that require a cushioned landing such as gymnastics.

3

Sports Injury Treatment and Rehabilitation

INTRODUCTION TO SPORTS INJURY MANAGEMENT

Sports injury management encompasses the entire process of treating a sports injury, right from the time the injury occurs through to the time the injured player is fully recovered and 110 per cent stronger and healthier than they were before the injury occurred. No, that is not a typo! The goal is 110 per cent because sports injury management should always aim to rehabilitate the injured area to the point where it is stronger after the injury than it was before the injury.

The types of sports injury that this management process is designed for are the soft tissue injuries, which are very common in most, if not all, sports. These injuries include sprains, strains, tears and bruises that affect the muscles, tendons, ligaments and joints – the soft tissues of the body.

Examples of common soft tissue injuries include hamstring tears, sprained ankles, pulled calf muscles, strained shoulder ligaments and corked thigh (bruised quadriceps). Remember, a sprain refers to a tear or rupture of the ligaments while a strain refers to a tear or rupture of the muscles or tendons.

The types of sports injury that this management process does not cover are injuries that affect the head, neck, face or spinal cord; injuries that involve shock, excessive bleeding, or bone fractures and breaks. The treatment needed for these types of injury is beyond the scope of the relatively simple soft tissue injuries that discussed here. Although this type of serious sports injury is rare, immediate medical attention must be sought.

Soft tissue sports injury management involves four phases:

1. First aid: the first three minutes
2. Treatment: the next three days
3. Rehabilitation: the next three weeks
4. Conditioning: the next three months

1. First Aid: The First Three Minutes

The first three minutes after an injury occurs are crucial. This is the time when an initial assessment of the injury is made and appropriate steps are taken to minimize trauma and prevent further damage. This is the first priority when treating any sports injury.

Before treating any injury, whether to yourself or someone else, first STOP and take account of what has occurred. Ask the questions: Is the area safe from other dangers? Is there a threat to life? Is the injury serious enough to seek emergency help?

Then, using the word **STOP,** as an acronym:

Stop: Stop the injured athlete from moving. Consider stopping the sport or game if necessary.
Talk: Ask questions like: What happened? How did it happen? What did it feel like? Where does it hurt? Have you injured this area before?
Observe: Look for signs like swelling, bruising, deformity and tenderness.
Prevent: Prevent further injury.

Next, make an assessment of the severity of the injury.

Is it a mild injury? Is it a bump or bruise that does not impair the athlete's physical performance? If so, play on. Provide a few words of encouragement and monitor the injury. Apply the treatment procedures described in Chapters 4–17 just to be on the safe side.

Is it a moderate injury? Is it a sprain, strain or severe bruise that impairs the athlete's ability to play on? If so, get the player off the field and apply the treatment procedures described in Chapters 4–17 as soon as possible.

Is it a severe injury? Does the injury affect the head, neck or face? Is there a possibility of spinal cord damage? Does it involve shock, excessive bleeding, or bone fractures and breaks? The treatment of these types of injury requires much more than simple soft tissue injury treatment. Seek professional help immediately.

Once a few moments have been taken to make sure the injury is not life threatening, it is time to start treating the injury. The sooner treatment is started, the more chance the injured athlete has of a full and complete recovery.

2. Treatment: The Next Three Days

Without a doubt, the most effective initial treatment for soft tissue injuries is the *RICER* regimen. This involves the application of (**R**) rest, (**I**) ice, (**C**) compression, (**E**) elevation and obtaining a (**R**) referral for appropriate medical treatment.

Where the RICER regimen has been used immediately after the occurrence of an injury, it has been shown to significantly reduce recovery time. RICER is the first and perhaps most important stage of injury rehabilitation, providing a basis for the complete recovery of injury.

When a soft tissue injury occurs there is inflammation around the injury site. Inflammation causes swelling that puts pressure on nerve endings and results in increased pain. It is exactly this process of inflammation, swelling and pain that the RICER regimen will help to alleviate. This will also limit tissue damage and aid the healing process.

Rest

It is important that the injured area be kept as still as possible. If necessary, support the injured area with a sling or brace. This will help to slow blood flow to the injured area and prevent any further damage.

Ice

This is by far the most important part. The application of ice will have the greatest effect on reducing inflammation, bleeding, swelling and pain. Apply ice as soon as possible after the injury has occurred.

How do you apply ice? Crushed ice in a plastic bag is usually best. However, blocks of ice, commercial cold packs and bags of frozen peas will all do fine. Even cold water from a tap is better than nothing at all.

When using ice, be careful not to apply it directly to the skin. This can cause ice burns and further skin damage. Wrapping the ice in a damp towel generally provides the best protection for the skin.

How long for and how often? There is much debate about this. The following are figures should be used as a rough guide, and then some advice from personal experience will be offered. The most common recommendation is to apply ice for 20 minutes every 2 hours for the first 48–72 hours.

These figures are a good starting point, but remember that they are only a guide. A number of precautions must be taken into account. Some people are more sensitive to cold than others. Children and elderly people have a lower tolerance to ice and cold, and people with circulatory problems are also more sensitive to ice.

The safest recommendation is that people use their own judgement when applying ice to the injured area. For some people, 20 minutes will be way too long. Others, especially well-conditioned athletes, can leave ice on for a lot longer.

The individual should make the decision as to how long the ice should stay on. People should apply ice for as long as it is comfortable. Obviously, there will be a slight discomfort from the cold, but as soon as pain or excessive discomfort is experienced it is time to remove the ice. It is much better to apply ice for 3–5 minutes a couple of times per hour than not at all.

Compression
Compression actually achieves two things. First, it helps to reduce bleeding and swelling around the injured area; second, it provides support for the injured area. Simply use a wide, firm, elastic compression bandage to cover the injured part. Bandage both above and below the injured area.

Elevation
Raise the injured area above the level of the heart whenever possible. This will further help to reduce the bleeding and swelling.

Referral
If the injury is severe enough, it is important that the injured athlete consult a professional physical therapist or a qualified sports doctor for an accurate diagnosis of the injury. With an accurate diagnosis, the athlete can then move on to a specific rehabilitation program to further reduce injury time.

A Word of Warning!
Before moving on, there are a few things that must be avoided during the first 48–72 hours after an injury. Be sure to avoid any form of heat at the injury site. This includes heat lamps, heat creams, spas, Jacuzzis and saunas. Avoid all movement and massage of the injured area. Also avoid excessive alcohol. All these things will increase the bleeding, swelling and pain of your injury. Avoid them at all costs.

3. Rehabilitation: The Next Three Weeks

When a muscle is torn or damaged it would be reasonable to expect the body to repair that damage with new muscle, or with new ligament if a ligament is damaged, and so on. In reality, this does not happen. The tear, or damage, is repaired with scar tissue.

When the RICER regimen is used immediately after a soft tissue injury occurs, it will limit the formation of scar tissue. However, some scar tissue will still be present.

This might not sound like a big deal, but anyone who has ever suffered a soft tissue injury will know how annoying it is to keep re-injuring that same old injury, over and over again. Untreated scar tissue is a major cause of re-injury, usually months after you thought that injury had fully healed.

Scar tissue is made from an inflexible, fibrous material called collagen. This fibrous material binds itself to damaged soft tissue fibres in an effort to draw the damaged fibres back together. What results is a bulky mass of fibrous scar tissue completely surrounding the injury site. In some cases it is even possible to see and feel this bulky mass under the skin.

When scar tissue forms around an injury site, it is never as strong as the tissue it replaces. It also has a tendency to contract and deform the surrounding tissues, so not only is the strength of the tissue diminished but flexibility of the tissue is also compromised.

So what does this mean for the athlete? First, it means a shortening of the soft tissues resulting in a loss of flexibility. Second, it means a weak spot has formed within the soft tissues which could easily result in further damage or re-injury.

The formation of scar tissue will result in a loss of strength and power. For a muscle to attain full power it must be fully stretched before contraction. Both the shortening effect and weakening of the tissues means that a full stretch and optimum contraction is no longer possible.

Getting Rid of Scar Tissue

To speed up the recovery process and remove or re-align the unwanted scar tissue, two vital treatments need to be initiated.

The first is commonly used by physical therapists (or physiotherapists) and primarily involves increasing the blood supply to the injured area. The aim is to increase the amount of oxygen and nutrients to the damaged tissues. Physical therapists accomplish by using a number of activities to stimulate the injured area. The most common methods used are ultrasound, TENS and heat.

Ultrasound uses high-frequency sound waves to stimulate the affected area. TENS (or Transcutaneous Electrical Nerve Stimulation) uses a light electrical pulse to give pain relief and increase blood flow. While heat in the form of a ray lamp or hot water bottle is very effective in stimulating blood flow to the damaged tissues.

The second treatment used to reduce unwanted scar tissue is deep tissue sports massage. While ultrasound and heat will help the injured area, they will not reduce scar tissue. Only massage will do that.

Either find someone who can massage the affected area or, if the injury is accessible, massage the damaged tissues yourself. Doing this yourself has the advantage of knowing just how hard and how deep you need to massage.

To start with, the area will be quite tender. Start with a light stroke and gradually increase the pressure until deep, firm strokes can be used. Massage in the direction of the muscle fibres and concentrate the most effort at the direct point of injury. Use the thumbs to get in as deep as possible to break down the scar tissue.

Recommended for improved soft tissue recovery is a remedy called Arnica. Arnica is extremely effective in treating soft tissue injuries such as sprains, strains and tears. It is available in a variety of forms such as massage gels and lotions.

Be sure to drink plenty of fluid during the injury rehabilitation process. The extra fluid will help to flush the waste products of injury and inflammation from the body.

Active Rehabilitation
As part of the rehabilitation phase the injured athlete will be required to do exercises and activities that will help to speed up the recovery process. Some people refer to this phase of the recovery process as the active rehabilitation phase because during this phase the athlete is responsible for the rehabilitation process.

The aim of this phase of the recovery is to regain all the fitness components that were lost during the injury process. Regaining flexibility, strength, power, muscular endurance, balance and coordination is the primary focus.

Without this phase of the rehabilitation process there is no hope of completely and permanently making a full recovery from your injury. Dornan and Dunn in *Sporting Injuries* (1988) emphasize the value of active rehabilitation:

"The injury symptoms will permanently disappear only after the patient has undergone a very specific exercise program, deliberately designed to stretch and strengthen and regain all parameters of fitness of the damaged structure or structures. Further, it is suggested that when a specific stretching program is followed, thus more permanently reorganizing the scar fibers and allowing the circulation to become normal, the painful symptoms will disappear permanently." (Ibid, 42-3)

The first point to make clear is how important it is to keep active. Often the advice from doctors and similar medical personnel will be simply to rest. This can be one of the worst things an injured athlete can do. Without some form of activity the injured area will not receive the blood flow it requires for recovery. An active circulation will provide both the oxygen and nutrients needed for the injury to heal.

Any form of gentle activity not only promotes blood circulation but also activates the lymphatic system. The lymphatic system is vital in clearing the body of toxins and waste products that accumulate in the tissues following a serious injury. Activity is the only way to activate the lymphatic system. Dornan and Dunn also support this approach:

"One does not need to wait for full anatomical healing before starting to retrain the muscle. The retraining can be started, gradually at first, during the healing period. This same principle applies also to ligamentous and tendon injuries." (Ibid, 39)

A Word of Warning!
Never do any activity that hurts the injured area or causes pain. Of course some discomfort may be experienced, but never push the injured area to the point where pain is felt. The recovery process is a long journey. Do not take a step backwards by overexerting the injured area. Be very careful with any activity. Pain is a warning sign: do not ignore it.

REGAINING THE FITNESS COMPONENTS

Now is the time to work on regaining the fitness components that were lost as a result of the injury. The main areas that need to be worked on are range of motion, flexibility, strength and coordination. Depending on the background of the athlete these elements should be the first priority. As the athlete starts to regain range of motion, strength, flexibility and coordination they can then start to work on the more specific areas of their chosen sport.

Range of Motion

Regaining a full range of motion is the first priority in this phase of the rehabilitation process. A full range of motion is extremely important as it lays the foundation for more intense and challenging exercises later in the active rehabilitation process.

While working through the initial stages of recovery the injury will begin to heal and the athlete should start to introduce some very gentle, movement-based exercises. First bending and straightening the injured area, then as this becomes more comfortable, starting to incorporate rotation exercises. Turn the injured area from side to side, and rotate clockwise and anti-clockwise. Dornan and Dunn emphasize:

> *"It is important that gentle stretching exercises be initiated early if normal flexibility is to be regained. For example, by actively stretching bruises of the thigh to their fullest pain-free extent, adhesion formation was limited and the thigh muscles were able to return to the pre-injury range of motion."* (Ibid, 39)

When these range of motion exercises can be performed relatively pain free, it is time to move on to the next phase of the active rehabilitation process.

Stretch and Strengthen

At this point increased intensity is added to the range of motion exercises. The aim here is to gradually re-introduce some flexibility and strength into the injured structures.

While attempting to increase the flexibility and strength of an injured area, be sure to approach it in a gradual, systematic way of lightly over-loading the injured area. Be careful not to over-do this type of training. Patience is required.

The use of machine weights can be very effective for improving the strength of an injured area as they provide a certain amount of stability to the joints and muscles as the athlete performs the rehabilitation exercises.

Another effective and relatively safe way to start is to begin with isometric exercises. These are exercise where the injured area does not move, yet force is applied and the muscles of the injured area are contracted.

For example: imagine sitting in a chair while facing a wall and then placing the ball of your foot against the wall. In this position you can push against the wall with your foot and at the same time keep your ankle joint from moving. The muscles contract but the ankle joint does not move. This is an isometric exercise.

It is also important during the active rehabilitation stage to introduce some gentle stretching exercises. These will help to further increase the range of motion and prepare the injured area for more strenuous activity.

Remember, while working on increasing the flexibility of an injured area it is important to increase the flexibility of the muscle groups around it. In the example above, these would include the calf muscles and the muscles of the shin.

Balance and Proprioception
Impaired balance and proprioception (the sense of movement and where the body is in space) commonly occur after soft tissue injury. This aspect of the rehabilitation process is often overlooked and is one of the main reasons why old injuries reoccur.

With soft tissue injury there is always a certain amount of damage to the nerve endings and pathways around the injured area. With less proprioceptive information, the brain has less information about the position of the joints and limbs around the injured area and the muscles are less able to work effectively. The results of a loss of proprioception include reduced balance, coordination, strength and stability. Local soft tissues are more vulnerable to strains and sprains, even to a reoccurrence of the same injury long after it was thought to have completely healed.

When improved flexibility and strength has returned to the injured area it is time to incorporate some balancing drills and exercises. Balancing exercises are important to help re-train the damaged nerves around the injured area. Start with simple balancing exercises such as walking along a straight line, or balancing on a beam. Progress to one-leg exercises such as balancing on one foot. Then try the same exercises with your eyes closed.

When comfortable with the above activities, try some of the more advanced exercises like wobble or rocker boards, Swiss balls, stability cushions and foam rollers.

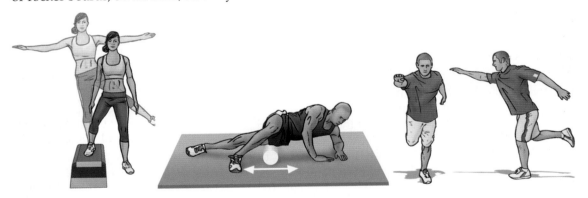

Examples of balance and proprioception exercises.

Final Preparation
This last part of the rehabilitation process will aim to return the individual to a pre-injury state. By the end of this process the injured area should be as strong, if not stronger, than it was before the injury occurred.

This is the time to incorporate some dynamic or explosive exercises to really strengthen up the injured area and improve proprioception. Start by working through all the exercises done during the previous stages of recovery, but with more intensity.

For example, if you were using light isometric exercises to help strengthen the Achilles tendon and calf muscles, start to apply more force, or start to use some weighted exercises.

Next, gradually incorporate some more intense exercises. Exercises that relate specifically to the athlete's chosen sport are a good place to start. Activities like skill drills and training exercises are a great way to gauge the fitness level and strength of the injured area.

To put the finishing touches to the recovery, incorporate simple plyometric drills. Plyometric exercises are explosive exercises that both lengthen and contract a muscle at the same time. These are called eccentric muscle contractions and are used in activities like jumping, hopping, skipping and bounding.

These activities are quite intense, so remember to always start off slowly and gradually apply more and more force. Do not get too excited and over-do it as patience and common sense are required.

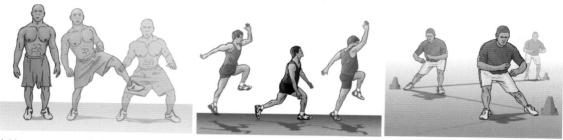

Add some more explosive exercises to aid recovery.

4. Conditioning: The Next Three Months

Where the above treatment procedures have been diligently applied, most soft tissue injuries will have completely healed. However, even though the initial injury may have healed and the athlete is able to return to normal activities, it is important to continue further strength and conditioning exercises to prevent a repeat of the initial injury.

The goal of the next three months is to identify the underlying causes or reasons why the injury occurred in the first place. Once identified, employ conditioning exercises or training aids that will help to prevent a reoccurrence of the initial injury.

To accomplish this phase effectively it is important to understand why sports injuries happen. Broadly speaking there are three main reasons why sports injuries occur. The first is accident, the second is overload and the third is biomechanical error.

Accident

Accidents include things like stepping into a pothole and spraining an ankle, tripping over and falling onto the shoulder or elbow, or being struck by sporting equipment. While there is little that can be done to prevent some accidents it is important to reduce risk as much as possible. A little common sense and diligently employing some of the prevention techniques described in Chapter 2 will help to minimize injuries caused by accidents.

Overload

Overload is common in sport and occurs when the structures within the body become fatigued and overworked. The structures then lose their ability to adequately perform their required task, which results in excessive strain (or overload) on other parts of the body.

For example, when the tensor fasciae latae muscle and iliotibial band, located in the thigh, become fatigued and overloaded, they lose their ability to adequately stabilize the entire leg. This in turn places stress on the knee joint, which results in pain and damage to the structures that make up the knee joint.

Most overload symptoms can be quickly reversed with adequate rest and relaxation. However, there are a number of things that will contribute to overload and should be avoided. They include:

- Exercising on hard surfaces like concrete
- Exercising on uneven ground
- Beginning an exercise program after a long lay-off period
- Increasing exercise intensity or duration too quickly
- Exercising in worn out or ill-fitting shoes
- Excessive uphill or downhill running

Biomechanical Error
Biomechanical errors are commonly responsible for many chronic injuries and occur when the structures within the body are not functioning as they should.

A common biomechanical error is muscle imbalance. This is where one muscle, or group of muscles, is either stronger or more flexible than its opposing muscles. This can occur on the left and right sides of the body or the front and back of the body.

For example, a right-handed baseball pitcher will commonly have overdeveloped shoulder and arm muscles on the right hand side compared with their left hand side. This can contribute to a pulling on the right of the spine and result in chronic pain in the shoulders, neck or back.

Another common example of muscle imbalance relates to hamstring strain. This can occur when the muscles of the quadriceps (thigh muscles) are strong and powerful while the hamstring muscles (located at the back of the thigh) are weak and inflexible.

Other biomechanical errors include:

- Leg length differences
- Tight or stiff muscles
- Foot structure problems such as flat feet
- Gait or running-style problems such as pronation or supination

Once the underlying cause or reason why the injury occurred has been identified, a conditioning program or training aid can be used to correct the problem. This may involve strength or flexibility exercises in the event of weak or tight muscles. It may involve orthotics or shoe inserts in the case of pronation, supination or leg length difference. Or it may involve the modification of the athlete's current training program to prevent overload.

4 Sports Injuries of the Skin

ANATOMY AND PHYSIOLOGY

The skin is the largest organ of the body. It has many functions. Its main role is to provide the body with a protective outer covering. The skin has three main layers: epidermis, dermis and subcutaneous layer.

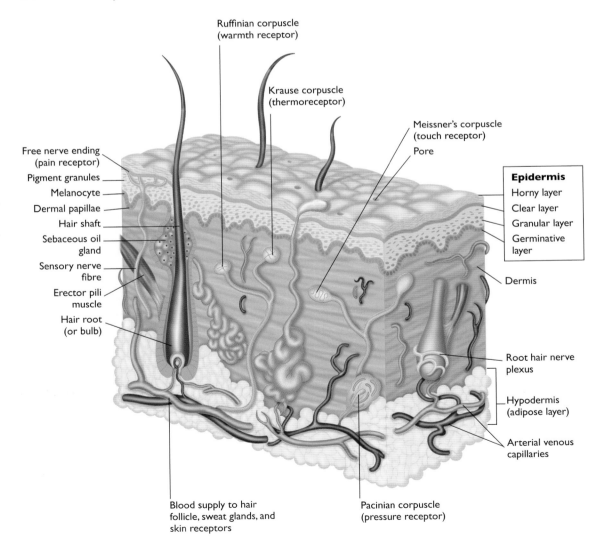

Ruffinian corpuscle (warmth receptor)

Krause corpuscle (thermoreceptor)

Meissner's corpuscle (touch receptor)

Pore

Free nerve ending (pain receptor)

Pigment granules

Melanocyte

Dermal papillae

Hair shaft

Sebaceous oil gland

Sensory nerve fibre

Erector pili muscle

Hair root (or bulb)

Epidermis
Horny layer
Clear layer
Granular layer
Germinative layer

Dermis

Root hair nerve plexus

Hypodermis (adipose layer)

Arterial venous capillaries

Blood supply to hair follicle, sweat glands, and skin receptors

Pacinian corpuscle (pressure receptor)

The epidermis is the outer covering of the skin and it is made up of many layers of cells. The thickness of these layers varies, depending on where it is on the body, ranging from the thickest parts, which are to be found on the palms of the hands and the soles of the feet to the thinnest on eyelids and lips. This layer has no blood vessels or nerve endings, but it is extremely sensitive to touch.

Cell renewal takes place in the epidermis. Living cells are formed in the basal layer and make their way through the layers of the epidermis and finally reach the corneal layer. While going through these layers, cells slowly die – their nuclei break down and they lose their fluid – and instead they fill with keratin. The outermost cells are constantly being worn away and replaced by the new cells growing up from below. This is a continuous process. It takes the skin approximately 28 days to completely renew itself.

The dermis is the thickest layer and is found beneath the epidermis. It supports and nourishes the epidermis. It is made up of dense connective tissue, which is tough, highly elastic and flexible. The tissue is highly sensitive and fibrous. The dermis also contains: collagen fibres, elastin fibres, blood vessels, lymph vessels, nerve supply, sensory nerves, motor nerves, hair follicles, sweat glands, sebaceous glands and erector pili muscles.

The subcutaneous layer is found below the dermis and its function is to produce and store fat. It consists of two layers, adipose tissue and areolar tissue. It is thicker in women than in men. As fat is a poor conductor of heat, this layer helps to reduce heat loss through the skin and so keeps the body warm. It also protects the nerves and blood vessels.

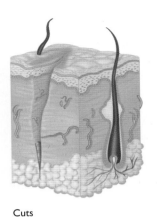

Cuts

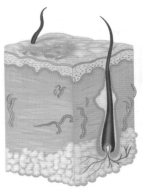

Abrasions

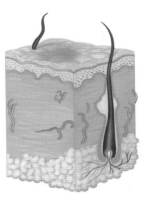

Chafing

CUTS, ABRASIONS, CHAFING

Skin cuts, abrasions and chafing are common afflictions among a broad variety of athletes. Such injuries involve superficial damage to the skin. The skin is broken in the case of cuts and sometimes in abrasions, while chafing is generally a surface phenomenon. While cuts are often caused by impact to the skin, chafing and abrasions are forms of superficial inflammatory dermatitis. Friction to skin leads to increased moisture and maceration. This causes a separation of keratin from the granular sublayer in the epidermis, sometimes resulting in an inflamed, oozing lesion. Generally, cuts, chafing and abrasions to the skin do not penetrate below the epidermis, unlike excoriation of the skin, which affects deeper layers. Cuts and abrasions can however cause bleeding, depending on the severity of injury. Deep abrasions can also produce scarring.

Cause of injury

Friction from athletic equipment, including padding and footwear. Fall onto a hard surface. Collision with another athlete. Friction of skin against clothing, combined with sweat and other moisture.

Signs and symptoms

Redness, pain and irritation. Itching or burning sensation. Bleeding.

Complications if left unattended

Skin injuries that are not properly treated can lead to potentially serious infections. Cuts, abrasions and chafing combined with moisture from sweat produce an ideal medium for bacteria and viruses. Infection is further encouraged when athletic equipment obstructs the skin.

Immediate treatment

Clean the affected area with soap and water, and dry thoroughly. Apply a topical steroid as needed. Bandage open wounds.

Rehabilitation and prevention

Cuts often result from sudden accidents such as falls and are not preventable. Wearing properly fitting clothing and footwear and drying areas prone to sweat with talcum or alum powders can minimize chafing and abrasions. Most chafing, cuts and abrasions of the skin heal naturally with minimal care and attention, providing infection is avoided.

Long-term prognosis

In more severe cases, performance may be detrimentally affected. Full recovery following healing of the skin is expected in most cases.

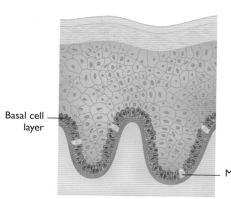

Basal cell layer

Melanocyte

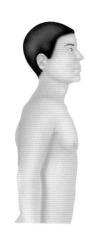

SUNBURN

Ultraviolet (UV) radiation from the sun can cause damage to the skin, typically sunburn which can range from mild to severe. All athletes engaged in outdoor sports are vulnerable to sunburn, particularly those performing at higher altitudes where atmospheric protection against UV rays is more limited. Skiers and mountaineers are hence at greater risk from sunburn than athletes closer to sea level. In the basal region of the skin's epidermis are dentritic cells known as melanocytes. Exposure to sunlight causes activity in these cells and the release of melanin, a pigment responsible for skin coloration. While gradual or less severe exposure produces tanning, excessive exposure causes damage to melanocytes, sometimes leading to a cancer of the skin known as melanoma.

Cause of injury
Excessive exposure to sunlight. Failure to cover exposed skin. Failure to apply sunscreen during extended exposure.

Signs and symptoms
Redness, pain and in severe cases blistering of the skin. Skin is hot to the touch.

Complications if left unattended
The most serious complication due to sunburn is melanoma, a potentially fatal cancer of the skin. Less severe complications involve damage to blood vessels, premature aging of the skin and loss of skin elasticity.

Immediate treatment
Get out of the sun as soon as possible. Cool baths as needed and topical moisturizers, including aloe vera.

Rehabilitation and prevention
Sunburn is usually treated without professional attention, providing it is not severe. Moisturizer may be applied to help prevent over-dryness and peeling of the skin, but the skin should not be covered with such products in the early phase of the injury while the body attempts to radiate heat. Prevent sunburn with Slip, Slop, Slap! Slip on a shirt, Slop on some sunscreen, and Slap on a hat.

Long-term prognosis
Most sunburn heals in a matter of days, though damaged layers may blister and peel away, with fresh skin replacing the dead layers. This new skin is particularly vulnerable to damage from the sun, and exposure should be avoided. Repeated overexposure to the sun increases the risk of skin cancer or melanoma.

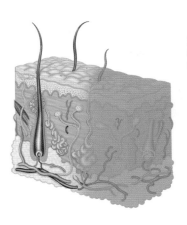

Freezing and crystallization causing cellular, and tissue death

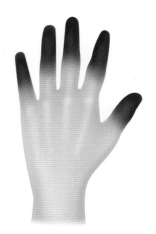

FROSTBITE

Athletes engaged in outdoor activities in cold weather are at risk of frostbite, an injury caused by a freezing of body tissue, resulting in damage to the skin and subcutaneous layers. Skiers and mountaineers are particularly prone to frostbite, which tends to affect exposed areas such as the nose and ears, as well as the body's extremities. Any athlete improperly protected against severe or prolonged exposure to low temperature is vulnerable.

Frostbite refers to the clinical condition in which water molecules within human tissue freeze and crystallize, causing cellular and tissue death. Early stages of frostbite are caused by ice formation in the extracellular tissue, causing damage to cell membranes and eventually cell and tissue death. Further freezing causes a shift in intracellular water to the extracellular space leading to dehydration and further, often irreversible damage.

Cause of injury
Prolonged exposure to the cold. Tissue getting wet and then freezing. Impeded blood flow in cold weather.

Signs and symptoms
Skin is white. Numbness or tingling, often in the hands and feet. Loose and blackened skin.

Complications if left unattended
Severe frostbite causes permanent damage to tissue and may result in gangrene, in some cases requiring amputation.

Immediate treatment
Immerse frozen areas in warm water or apply warm compresses. Analgesics for pain.

Rehabilitation and prevention
Thawing of serious frostbite must be done carefully. Avoid rubbing the affected area. If blistering has occurred, the area should be wrapped in a sterile bandage. Do not thaw areas at risk of refreezing as more serious tissue damage may result. Frostbite is prevented by avoiding prolonged exposure to the cold and activities at extremely low temperatures.

Long-term prognosis
Mild to moderate frostbite may leave the athlete at some increased risk for future cold sensitivity and re-injury. Severe frostbite can cause irreversible damage requiring amputation, though such injuries are usually restricted to those engaged in high-altitude sports, particularly mountaineering.

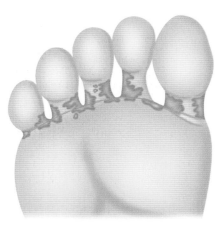

ATHLETE'S FOOT (TINEA PEDIS)

Athlete's foot is caused by a fungal infection of the foot produced by a class of parasites of the skin known as dermatophytes. The affliction is common among athletes and thrives in moist conditions produced by sweat. The ailment causes a red, itchy rash-like condition on the feet and may be spread to others. The most common form of the condition is known as chronic interdigital athlete's foot.

The site most commonly affected is between the spaces of the fourth and fifth toes where it causes irritation, maceration, fissures and scaling of the outer layer of skin. Infection can spread to the dorsal and plantar surfaces of the foot and into the nails, where it starts as a yellowing of the distal margin and/or along the edge of a nail. The fungi responsible are plant organisms (tinea pedis), and bacteria may produce secondary infections which worsens the symptoms.

Cause of injury
Excessive sweating. Contagious transmission. Failure to wash and properly dry the feet.

Signs and symptoms
Reddened, cracked and peeling skin. Itching, burning, stinging sensation. Bad odour.

Complications if left unattended
Without proper care, athlete's foot can worsen, deepening the fissures in the skin, spreading across the foot surface, affecting the soles and toenails and occasionally spreading to the palms of the hands as well. The burning and itching sensation increases along with odour, and the risk of spreading the infection to others increases.

Immediate treatment
Wash and thoroughly dry the feet. Apply topical antifungal medication.

Rehabilitation and prevention
Athlete's foot is a common occurrence, affecting 70 per cent of the population at various times. Generally, it responds well with minimal care – washing the feet often and seeing that they are thoroughly dried and, whenever possible, kept dry during the day. If the nail is infected the condition can be difficult to treat, requiring aggressive care. Chronically affected toenails may need to be removed by a podiatrist.

Long-term prognosis
Most cases of athlete's foot are resolved with proper hygiene and application of anti-fungal medication. More severe cases may require a long-term regimen of oral medication and nail removal to fully resolve the issue.

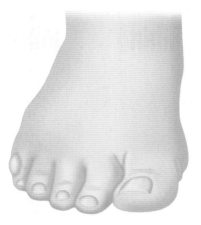

BLISTERS

Blisters are a common injury in many sports where the skin encounters friction, either from footwear (during running events, skating, skiing, etc.) or sporting apparatus, for example, in gymnastics, baseball or racket events. Small, fluid-filled bubbles or vesicles form on the skin in response to friction. Generally, the fluid is clear but occasionally bleeding into the blister causes red or blue discoloration.

Blisters occur when there is a separation of the epidermis from the dermal layer of skin or a separation within the multiple layers of the epidermis itself. Serum, lymph, blood or extracellular fluid fills the space between layers. Thin, translucent walls are formed and the area swells and may become sensitive or painful.

Cause of injury
Friction to feet from running sports. Friction to fingers and palms from golf clubs, tennis rackets, etc. Friction to hands from acrobatics and gymnastics activities.

Signs and symptoms
Raised, translucent bubbles of skin in the area of wear. Pain, stinging and sensitivity at the site of injury. Leakage of fluid should the blister be disturbed.

Complications if left unattended
If athletic activities are continued without attention to the blisters they may become torn, resulting in further irritation to the skin and pain. Improperly treated blisters also run the risk of infection as the open wound is a point of entry for bacteria and other germs.

Immediate treatment
Wash the blister(s) gently with soap and warm water. If needed, carefully drain fluid. Cover with sterile bandage.

Rehabilitation and prevention
Blisters generally heal with minimal care and proper attention, providing no infection has occurred. Properly fitting socks and footwear can help avoid blisters among runners. Other athletes may chalk their hands to lessen blister-causing friction, particularly in the case of gymnasts. Proper attention to athletic technique may also help minimize blisters.

Long-term prognosis
Blisters heal in a few days to a week, providing there is no serious infection. Until they have healed however, blisters can sometimes interfere with performance due to pain and discomfort.

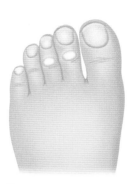

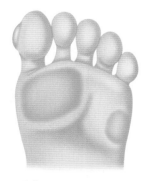

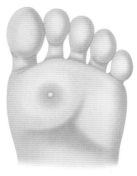

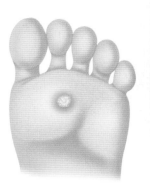

Corns *Calluses* *Plantar wart (verrucae)*

CORNS, CALLUSES, PLANTAR WARTS (VERRUCAE)

Corns and calluses are both caused by friction and pressure – in athletes this is often due to pressure from shoes or weightbearing. Plantar warts (verrucae) result from the human papilloma virus (HPV).

A corn is a horny thickening of the stratum corneum of the skin of the toes. A callus is a localized thickening of the horny layer of the epidermis due to physical trauma.

Calluses often occur on weightbearing areas of the plantar surface (sole) of the foot, and may result from abnormal alignment of the metatarsal bones in the ball of the foot. Corns and calluses may have a deeper central core, or nucleation, which tends to be extremely tender, and are characterized by a gradual thickening and toughening of the skin, eventually leading to irritation.

Warts are the result of an infection by the highly contagious HPV. Warts are epidermal lesions with a horny surface. They occur on many parts of the body, including the soles of the feet, where they are known as plantar warts or verrucae.

Cause of injury
Repeated friction. Weightbearing. Contagious transmission (plantar warts).

Signs and symptoms
Thickened skin where prominent bones press against the shoe (corns). Tough or thickened skin on the soles of the feet (calluses). Raised, disfigured areas of skin on the ball, heel and bottom of the big toe (plantar warts).

Complications if left unattended
In the case of corns and calluses the condition may worsen, eventually causing pain requiring medical attention. Warts can spread to other body areas as well as to others.

Immediate treatment
In the case of corns and calluses, alleviate the source of pressure on the foot. In the case of plantar warts, apply anti-viral medication and cover the area.

Rehabilitation and prevention
Corns and calluses are injuries directly related to pressure on the foot and are resolved by addressing the source of pressure, whether due to footwear or weightbearing. Corns and calluses respond well to treatment, while warts have a tendency to recur. Proper athletic footwear and attention to technique can help prevent corns and calluses while verrucae may be prevented with attention to hygiene and avoidance of environments prone to the HPV.

Long-term prognosis
Corns and calluses are usually a minor inconvenience to the athlete and clear up thoroughly once their source has been addressed. When they are a source of pain or continuing discomfort, they may be addressed through cryotherapy, excision, laser surgery or other methods.

5 Sports Injuries of the Head and Neck

THE HEAD

The cranium (Greek: kranion) is made up of eight large flat bones comprising two pairs plus four single bones. These form a box-like container that houses the brain. These bones are:

Frontal: which forms the forehead, the bony projections under the eyebrows and the superior part of the orbit of each eye.

Parietal: a pair of bones that form most of the superior and lateral walls of the cranium. They meet in the midline at the sagittal suture, and meet with the frontal bone at the coronal suture.

Temporal: a pair of bones that lie inferior to the parietal bones. There are three important markings on the temporal bone: (a) the styloid process, a sharp, needle-like projection to which many of the neck muscles attach; (b) the zygomatic process, a thin bridge of bone that joins with the zygomatic bone just above the mandible; (c) the mastoid process, a rough projection posterior and inferior to the styloid process (just behind the lobe of the ear).

Occipital: the most posterior bone of the cranium. It forms the floor and back wall of the skull, and joins the parietal bones anteriorly at the lambdoid suture. In the base of the occipital bone is a large opening, the foramen magnum, through which the spinal cord passes to connect with the brain. To each side of the foramen magnum are the occipital condyles which rest on the first vertebra of the spinal column (the atlas).

Sphenoid: a butterfly-shaped bone that spans the width of the skull and forms part of the floor of the cranial cavity. Parts of the sphenoid can be seen forming part of the eye orbits and the lateral part of the skull.

Ethmoid: a single bone in front of the sphenoid bone and below the frontal bone. Forms part of nasal septum and superior and medial conchae.

The Facial Bones

Fourteen bones compose the face, twelve of which are paired. The main bones of the face are:

Nasal: a pair of small rectangular bones that form the bridge of the nose (the lower part of the nose is made up of cartilage).

Zygomatic: a pair of bones commonly known as the cheekbones. They also form a large portion of the lateral walls of the eye orbits.

Maxillae: the two maxillary bones fuse to form the upper jaw. The upper teeth are embedded in the maxillae.

Mandible: the lower jawbone is the strongest bone in the face. It joins the temporal bones on each side of the face, forming the only freely movable joints in the skull. The horizontal part of the mandible, or the body, forms the chin. Two upright bars of bone, or rami, extend from the body to connect the mandible with the temporal bone. The lower teeth are embedded in the mandible.

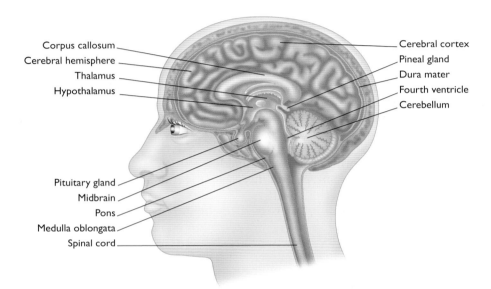

a)

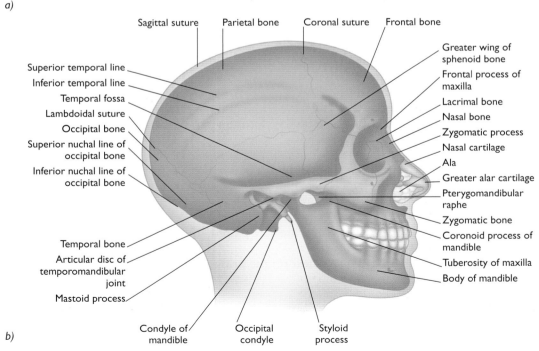

b)

The head, lateral view, and b) the skull, lateral view.

Teeth

Teeth are hard, calcified structures set in the alveolar processes of the mandible and maxilla. Each tooth consists of a crown, a neck and a root. The solid part includes dentin, which forms most of the tooth; enamel, which covers the crown; and cementum covering the root. In the centre is the soft pulp containing arteries, veins, and lymphatic and nerve tissue.

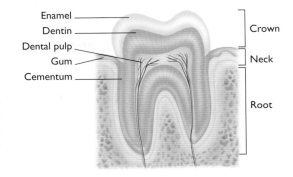

Eyes

The eyes, among the body's most delicate structures, are protected by design from injury. The eyeball is a large sphere, and is recessed in a socket surrounded by a strong, bony ridge, with the segment of a smaller sphere, the cornea, in front. The eyelids can close quickly, protecting the eyeball from foreign objects. Furthermore, the eye is designed to withstand some impact without serious damage.

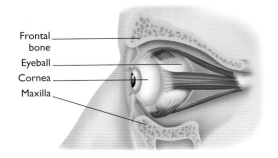

Ears

The ear is the organ responsible for hearing, also playing a critical role in balance (equilibrium). Injury to the ear can affect either or both of these senses. The outer ear consists of the outer cartilage (pinna) and the auditory canal. The middle ear consists of the tympanic membrane (or eardrum); the auditory ossicles or bones of the ear; the middle ear cavity and the Eustachian tube.

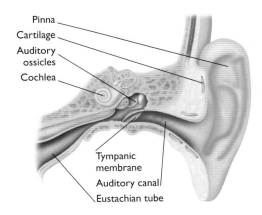

Nose

The nose is comprised of bone and cartilage. The nasal septum is often injured in sports. It consists of the vomer, a perpendicular plate of the ethmoid, and the quadrangular cartilage. A pair of protrusions from the frontal bones and the ascending processes of the maxilla complete the bony component, while the upper lateral and lower lateral cartilages, as well as the cartilaginous septum, make up the non-bony portion.

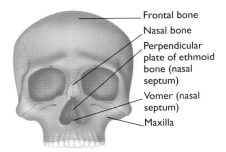

THE NECK

The cervical spine (neck) is made up of seven vertebrae, which begin at the base of the skull (C1) and angle downward slightly as they reach the chest region and connect with the thoracic vertebrae. Muscles running from the rib cage and clavicle (collarbone) to the cervical vertebrae, jaw and skull appear on the front or anterior cervical area. The posterior cervical muscles cover the bones along the back of the spine and make up the bulk of the tissues on the back of the neck.

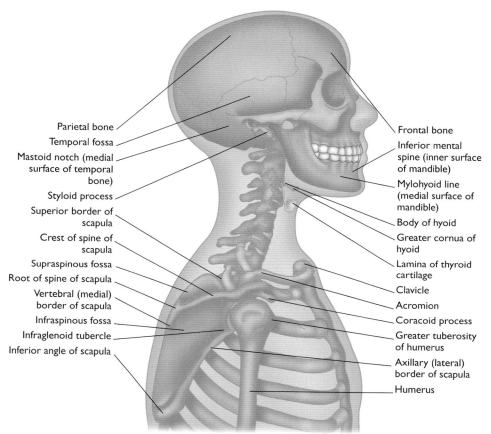

Parietal bone
Temporal fossa
Mastoid notch (medial surface of temporal bone)
Styloid process
Superior border of scapula
Crest of spine of scapula
Supraspinous fossa
Root of spine of scapula
Vertebral (medial) border of scapula
Infraspinous fossa
Infraglenoid tubercle
Inferior angle of scapula

Frontal bone
Inferior mental spine (inner surface of mandible)
Mylohyoid line (medial surface of mandible)
Body of hyoid
Greater cornua of hyoid
Lamina of thyroid cartilage
Clavicle
Acromion
Coracoid process
Greater tuberosity of humerus
Axillary (lateral) border of scapula
Humerus

The head and neck, lateral view.

The brachial plexus is a collection of nerves supplying the upper limb. They exit the cervical vertebrae, extending to peripheral structures including muscles and the skin (transmitting motor and sensory nerve impulses). Cervical nerve roots within the brachial plexus send fibres to the shoulder, the arm and forearm, the elbow, wrist, hand and fingers.

Between the cervical vertebrae, intervertebral discs absorb shock, facilitate movement and provide support for the spinal column. Such discs consist of a central region or nucleus pulposus and a surrounding annulus fibrosis separating each segmental vertebra between from C2 to T1 (the first thoracic vertebra). (Only ligaments and joint capsules exist between C1 and C2).

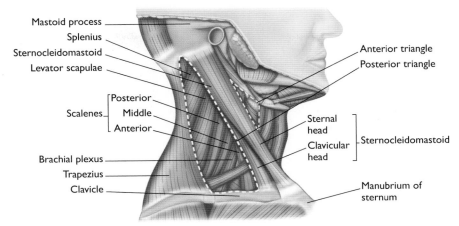

The neck muscles, lateral view.

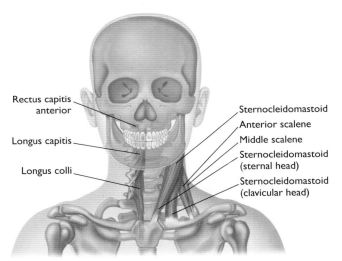

The neck muscles, anterior view.

Most anterior neck muscles flex the cervical spine, bringing the head downward. When standing or sitting, gravity assists and the heavy weight of the head helps. This can cause weakness in the antagonist muscles, the extensors, if it becomes habitual. The strong pull of the large sternocleidomastoid muscle, along with small deeper muscles (longus colli, longus capitis and rectus capitis anterior) can pull the head down as well as support it.

The extensors on the back of the neck must concentrically contract to lift the head. Straightening the upper spine is work for many muscles: the splenii, scalenes, upper erector spinae, semispinalis, deep posterior muscles and obliquus capitis, even the trapezius. These muscles also do either lateral flexion (along with the levator scapula) or rotation of the neck, so they are easy to strengthen because of the many actions they perform.

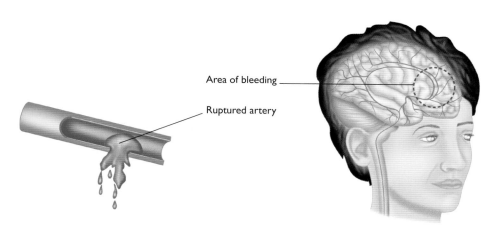

Area of bleeding

Ruptured artery

HEAD CONCUSSION, CONTUSION, HAEMORRHAGE, FRACTURE

Traumas to the head are amongst the most serious injuries facing an athlete. Among these are: concussion, involving sudden acceleration of the head; contusion or bruising of the brain tissue; haemorrhage or bleeding inside the skull, and fracture or breaking of the bones of the skull. Athletes engaged in contact sports such as boxing, football, rugby, lacrosse and hockey are the most vulnerable to such injuries.

If the force is sufficient, bones of the skull can fracture, sometimes impinging on brain tissue. Bleeding or haemorrhage inside the skull can occur (with or without fracture). If a blood vessel lying between the skull and the brain ruptures it may form a clot or haematoma, which may press on the underlying brain tissue. A clot forming between the skull and the brain's protective covering or dura mater is known as an epidural haematoma while a clot below the dura is known as a subdural haematoma. Haemorrhage in deeper layers may cause a contusion or bruising to the brain tissue.

Cause of injury
Forceful collision with another athlete during contact sports. Serious fall with impact to the head. Trauma from blow in boxing.

Signs and symptoms
Loss of consciousness. Confusion and memory loss. Shock.

Complications if left unattended
Head injuries require immediate medical attention. Failure to seek prompt, professional care can result in permanent brain damage and, in more severe cases, fatality.

Immediate treatment
Immobilize patient (with head and shoulders raised) in a quiet place. Staunch the flow of blood if necessary and seek immediate medical care.

Rehabilitation and prevention
Rehabilitation from head injuries varies widely depending on the nature and extent. Even mild concussions result in a post-concussion syndrome in many patients, which can persist for six months to a year. More serious injuries can cause a broad array of permanent symptoms. Helmets or other appropriate headgear in sports where the skull is vulnerable help prevent such injuries.

Long-term prognosis
Prognosis for a head injury may not be fully known for months or, in some cases, years. In the case of a mild injury, the prognosis is generally good, though symptoms including headache, dizziness and amnesia may persist. Blood clots, haemorrhaging and fractures of the skull often require surgery.

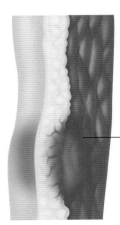
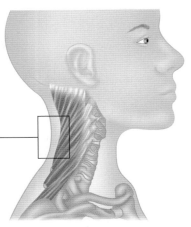

NECK STRAIN, FRACTURE, CONTUSION

Injuries to the neck can be serious, particularly in the case of broken or fractured vertebrae. Neck strains are less serious and far more common, and involve injury to the muscles or tendons of the neck. Contusions are bruises to the skin and underlying tissue of the neck, usually the result of a direct blow.

Cause of injury
Sudden twisting of the neck. Serious fall. Direct blow to the neck, in the case of contusion.

Signs and symptoms
Head, neck and shoulder pain. Crackling sensation in the neck. Loss of neck strength and mobility.

Complications if left unattended
Injuries to the neck are potentially serious and deserve prompt medical attention. Long-term paralysis, loss of motion and coordination, calcification and osteoporosis are possible side-effects. In the case of fracture, the injury can lead to paraplegia and is also sometimes fatal.

Immediate treatment
Immobilization to protect the spinal cord. Analgesics for pain.

Rehabilitation and prevention
For neck strains, immobilization for a period of weeks with a brace may be recommended. In cases of fracture, the broken vertebrae may be surgically pinned together with screws and the patient may be placed in a neck cast. Physical therapy following healing will attempt to re-establish range of motion, flexibility and strength. Helmets or other athletic headgear as well as attention to proper technique can help prevent some neck injuries.

Long-term prognosis
Outcomes for neck injury vary widely depending on the nature and severity. In cases of fracture, the prognosis is generally worse with injuries occurring higher up the cervical spine.

Neck strains and contusions are far less serious and their outcome given proper treatment and rehabilitation is usually good. Severe strains in which the muscle–tendon–bone attachment is ruptured may require surgical repair.

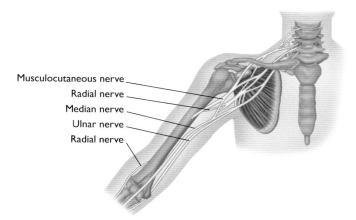

Musculocutaneous nerve
Radial nerve
Median nerve
Ulnar nerve
Radial nerve

CERVICAL NERVE STRETCH SYNDROME

Cervical nerve stretch syndrome, also referred to as burner syndrome, results from the stretching (or compression) of the brachial plexus, a complex of nerves in the lower neck and shoulder area. The injury is common in contact sports including hockey, football, wrestling and rugby. Sports injuries to the brachial plexus are characterized by a burning sensation that radiates down an upper extremity. Symptoms may last anywhere from two minutes to two weeks.

Cause of injury
Blow to the head or shoulder, especially in a football tackle. Ear-to-shoulder bending with rotation (causing compression of cervical nerves). Hyperextension of the neck.

Signs and symptoms
Severe, burning pain, radiating from the neck to the arm and/or fingers. Paraesthesia or numbness, tingling, pricking, burning or creeping sensation of the skin. Muscle weakness.

Complications if left unattended
Burning and stinging symptoms will persist and often worsen. Further damage to peripheral nerves can result should the injury be ignored. Symptoms may also indicate spinal cord injury, with potentially serious complications.

Immediate treatment
Ice and immobilize the neck region. Anti-inflammatory medication and analgesics for pain.

Rehabilitation and prevention
Rehabilitation for cervical nerve stretch syndrome usually entails physical therapy. Following a healing phase, therapy seeks to improve cervical range of motion and to strengthen cervical muscles, with particular attention to the muscles supporting the injured brachial plexus nerve. Proper protective gear, appropriate technique and upper-extremity strength training can help prevent the injury.

Long-term prognosis
Prognosis for the injury is generally good, though some athletes develop a chronic form of the condition and a high rate of re-injury has also been noted. In rare cases, nerve injury requires microsurgery to repair nerve damage.

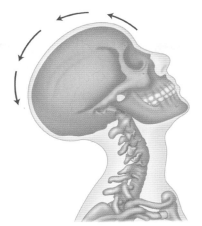

WHIPLASH (NECK STRAIN)

Whiplash injury occurs when there is sudden flexion and/or extension of the neck, usually when the athlete is struck from behind during contact sports, and the head is rapidly thrown both forward and backward. Soft tissues of the neck including intervertebral discs, ligaments, cervical muscles and nerve roots may be injured, producing neck pain, stiffness and loss of mobility.

The hips, back and trunk are the first body segments and joints to experience movement during a whiplash. Forward motion in these structures is accompanied by upward motion, which acts to compress the cervical spine. This combined motion causes the head to move backward into extension, producing tension where the lower cervical segment extends and the upper cervical segment flexes. With this movement of the cervical vertebrae, the anterior structures are separated and posterior components including facet joints are severely compressed.

Cause of injury
Tackle from behind, e.g. football. Sharp collision with another athlete or piece of equipment. Blow to the head, e.g. boxing.

Signs and symptoms
Pain and stiffness in the neck, shoulder or between the shoulder blades. Ringing in the ears or blurred vision. Irritability and fatigue.

Complications if left unattended
Left untreated, whiplash injury can produce chronic symptoms of pain, inflexibility and loss of movement, along with the continuation or worsening of associated symptoms of fatigue, sleep loss, memory and concentration loss and depression. Symptoms may also suggest more serious injury to the spinal vertebrae with potentially serious consequences.

Immediate treatment
The RICER regimen. Immobilization with a cervical collar.

Rehabilitation and prevention
The neck will usually be immobilized with some form of brace, though early movement is usually encouraged to prevent stiffening. Low-impact strength and flexibility training and rehabilitation should follow complete healing of the tendons, discs and ligaments. Risk of whiplash may be minimized with protective gear as well as a thorough warm-up routine, though prevention in rough contact sports may not be guaranteed.

Long-term prognosis
The long-term prognosis for most whiplash injuries is good, given adequate care, though symptoms may persist and the neck may be prone to re-injury.

WRYNECK (TORTICOLLIS)

Wryneck or torticollis is a painful neck injury that usually follows a sudden rotational movement of the head. Nerves in the neck are compressed, resulting in muscle spasms, accompanying pain and loss of movement. While irritation of the discs of the cervical spine, or disc prolapse (rupturing), can lead to the condition, sudden injury, as during sports activity, is usually the result of compression of the nerves in the neck or a sprain of one of the facet joints. Typically the neck is frozen in one position, often rotated to one side and bent forward by the contraction of the cervical muscles.

Many sports can cause the injury. Symptoms are often first experienced in the morning on waking. Immediate-onset torticollis is usually facet joint related; slow-onset torticollis (as after sleep) is often disc related.

Cause of injury
Sudden rotation of the head in contact sports. A fall that causes a sudden torsion in the neck. Direct blow to the head, causing sudden twisting.

Signs and symptoms
Pain and stiffness. Loss of motion. Neck may be stuck or frozen in one position.

Complications if left unattended
Wryneck can worsen, in some cases becoming chronic if ignored. The condition may indicate damage to the cervical vertebrae, cervical discs or associated nerves and joints, requiring medical attention.

Immediate treatment
Immobilization of the injured neck with a brace or supportive cervical collar. Anti-inflammatory medication and ice to reduce swelling.

Rehabilitation and prevention
It is critical to determine the cause of the injury and rule out serious underlying conditions requiring surgery or major medical intervention. Following this, a physical therapist may use an infrared heat lamp as well as massage of the cervical muscles in order to restore range of motion in the injured neck. Protective headgear, upper body and neck strength training and attention to proper athletic technique may help reduce the likelihood of this injury.

Long-term prognosis
Wryneck usually resolves in a week or less, though the painful spasms can be temporarily debilitating. While a chronic form of the condition exists, for most a full recovery can be expected, barring more serious underlying conditions.

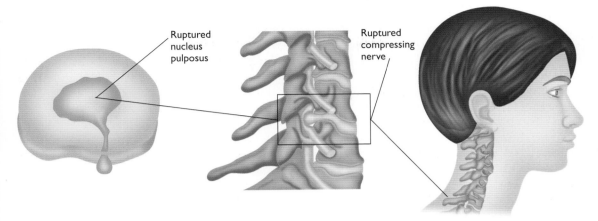

Ruptured nucleus pulposus

Ruptured compressing nerve

CERVICAL DISC INJURY (ACUTE CERVICAL DISC DISEASE)

Cervical discs are shock-absorbing pads of tissue cushioning the bones of the cervical spine. A variety of injuries to these discs can cause pain and hamper movement and flexibility of the neck. Herniated discs occur when the gel-like substance of the nucleus pulposus bulges or leaks from the disc's interior, following a split or rupture to the disc. This substance can then exert pressure on the spinal cord or nerves of the cervical spine. Disc degeneration and/or herniation (disc rupture) can cause injury to the spinal cord or nerve roots. Bulging discs occur when the disc extends outside its normal boundary but no rupture or tear has occurred.

Cause of injury
Disc degeneration and loss of elasticity. Repetitive stress, particularly from excessive or improper weightlifting. Sudden, forceful trauma to the cervical vertebrae.

Signs and symptoms
Tingling and weakness. Numbness or pain in the neck, shoulder, arm or hand. Loss of strength in the muscles supplied by the affected spinal nerve.

Complications if left unattended
Herniated or slipped discs can impinge on the spinal cord, an extremely delicate structure. Even minor damage to the spinal cord can be serious and is generally not reparable. Ignoring cervical disc injuries can lead to further degeneration and associated pain and mobility loss.

Immediate treatment
Discontinue activity causing stress to cervical vertebrae and discs. Rest, ice and use of anti-inflammatory medication.

Rehabilitation and prevention
For most disc injuries, a conservative course of treatment is undertaken. The neck may be immobilized for a period in a cervical collar during healing. Physical therapy includes mobilizing, stretching, strengthening and proprioceptive exercises and sometimes efforts to adjust posture. Upper body exercise may help prevent disc hardening and degeneration, while strengthening supporting muscles will lower the risk of rupture.

Long-term prognosis
The majority of disc injuries improve without recourse to surgery. Most athletes can expect a full return to normal performance following rest and rehabilitation, though symptoms of the injury occasionally recur and degenerated discs are prone to re-injury.

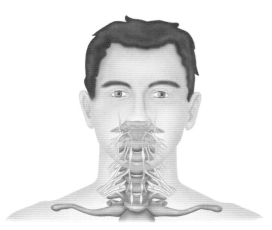

PINCHED NERVE (CERVICAL RADICULITIS)

Nerves controlling the shoulder, arm and hand originate in the spinal cord in the neck. Inflammation or compression of one of these structures is known as a pinched nerve or cervical radiculitis and results in pain, weakness and loss of movement.

Cervical radiculitis occurs when a disc from one of the cervical vertebrae presses against one of the spinal nerves emerging from the spinal cord. Such nerves branch to numerous areas of the body and symptoms may radiate from the source along the nerve to areas where the nerve travels. Depending on the affected disc, pain may occur in the hand, arm, neck or shoulder.

Cause of injury

Herniated disc pressing on a nerve. Irritation of the nerve due to repetitive stress. Bone spurs or degenerating vertebrae impinging on a nerve.

Signs and symptoms

Pain, weakness and loss of movement in the neck. Numb fingers. Weakness in the hand, arm, shoulder or chest.

Complications if left unattended

Inflammation and pain associated with pinched nerves may continue or worsen should the source of the injury not be addressed. The nerve may become permanently damaged through continued pressure and stress, and the condition may point to other (potentially serious) underlying injuries to the vertebrae or spinal cord.

Immediate treatment

Cease activity stressful to the cervical spine. Rest, ice, analgesics and anti-inflammatory medication.

Rehabilitation and prevention

Given proper treatment, the prognosis for cervical radiculitis is generally good. Mild cases usually respond to physical therapy in conjunction with medications such as non-steroidal anti-inflammatory drugs (NSAIDs) or steroids. Following healing, a program of physical therapy and flexibility/strengthening exercises can help restore the athlete's former condition. Attention to proper technique, particularly during weight training/weightlifting can help prevent pinched nerve injury.

Long-term prognosis

Most cervical pinched nerve injuries resolve themselves without serious medical intervention. More serious or prolonged cases may require surgery to relieve compression of the nerve root.

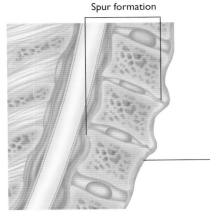

Spur formation

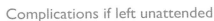

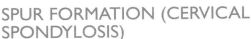

SPUR FORMATION (CERVICAL SPONDYLOSIS)

Cervical spondylosis is a chronic degenerative condition of the cervical spine and the intervertebral discs. Aging and repetitive stress cause discs to become drier, thinner and less elastic. When the surrounding ligaments become less supportive, the vertebrae develop bone spurs, or osteophytes, which are bony projections that form along joints.

Bone spurs are the body's attempt to stabilize degenerative joints and are often associated with arthritis or advanced wear and tear such as that experienced by athletes who play high-impact sports such as rugby. Such spurs themselves can rub against nearby nerves or occasionally on the spinal cord, causing pain, neurological symptoms and limitations in joint motion.

Cause of injury
Repetitive wear on cervical vertebrae. Excessive or improper weightlifting. Bulging or herniated cervical disc.

Signs and symptoms
Neck pain radiating to shoulders and arms. Loss of balance. Headaches radiating to the back of the head.

Complications if left unattended
Cervical spondylosis is a common cause of spinal cord dysfunction in older adults. If the condition isn't treated, the injury may progress and become permanent. Bone spurs or herniated discs can impinge and put pressure on the roots of one or more nerves of the spinal cord in the neck, producing tingling, burning, weakness or numbness in the arms or hands. Displaced spurs can also float in the system, periodically interfering with joints.

Immediate treatment
Neck brace or cervical collar to help limit neck motion. NSAIDs.

Rehabilitation and prevention
Less serious cases of cervical spondylosis respond to exercises prescribed by a physical therapist aimed at strengthening and stretching neck muscles. Low-impact aerobic exercises including walking or swimming may also help. While age-related spondylosis may be difficult to prevent, minimizing high-impact activity, engaging in upper body training and attention to posture may help avoid the injury.

Long-term prognosis
Mild cases of cervical spondylosis respond well after immobilization of the area and appropriate physical therapy. More serious cases may require injections of corticosteroids between the vertebral facet joints or, in some cases, surgery to remove bone spurs, particularly if they have broken off from larger sections of bone to become loose bodies.

TEETH

Injury to the teeth is a particular risk for athletes involved in sports where a projectile such as a ball or puck can strike the player's face. Such sports include hockey, lacrosse and football. The most common injuries of this sort are a fractured, displaced or avulsed (knocked out) tooth. Injuries to the teeth often accompany other head and neck injuries, including fractured facial bones, concussions, abrasions, bruises, soft tissue lacerations with bleeding and jaw-joint problems.

Teeth can be chipped or in some cases knocked out altogether, given sufficient force from a bat or ball. The avulsed tooth runs the risk of being rejected by the body as a foreign object and should therefore be cleaned and replaced firmly in its socket as soon after the injury as possible.

Cause of injury
Teeth struck with a ball, puck or other projectile. Direct blow in boxing. Teeth struck by equipment including bats, sticks, racquets, etc.

Signs and symptoms
Mouth pain. Loose teeth. Bleeding from the mouth.

Complications if left unattended
Injury to the teeth should receive prompt medical attention. Swallowing a tooth after injury is a danger, as is infection in the mouth if the injury is not properly cleaned and attended to.

Immediate treatment
If the tooth has been knocked out, wash in saline and replace firmly in the socket. Rinse mouth and use analgesics and ice for pain relief.

Rehabilitation and prevention
Rehabilitation from injury to the teeth is dependent on the nature and severity. Chipped or fractured teeth can be repaired and bonded by a dentist and lost teeth replaced. The athlete should refrain from activities that put the teeth at risk until thorough healing has been accomplished. Use of a mouth guard, particularly a custom-fitted one, helps protect the teeth during high-risk and contact sports.

Long-term prognosis
Most injuries to the teeth, while painful, do not threaten an athlete's career or future performance, particularly provided they are given proper medical and dental attention. A knocked out tooth has a good prognosis for replanting, providing this is done within the first thirty minutes of the injury. After more than two hours the prognosis is poor for tooth replacement due to rejection of the tooth and re-absorption of the root.

EYE

Injuries to the eye are always potentially serious. Many sports entail risk to the eyes, particularly those involving a ball, puck, stick, bat or racquet or other apparatus, such as a fencing foil. Basketball, hockey, netball and baseball cause the most eye injuries, while sports carrying a low risk of injury to the eye include track and field, swimming, gymnastics and cycling. Exposure of the eyes to excess ultraviolet (UV) radiation can also cause damage, necessitating protection of the eyes in sports like skiing and mountaineering. Even minor eye injuries can impair vision and complications can result in visual deficit or loss.

Cause of injury
Blunt trauma to the eye from equipment or direct contact, e.g. wrestling. Penetrating injury to the eye. Radiation damage due to sun overexposure.

Signs and symptoms
Blurred or absent vision. Pain or sensitivity in the eye. Obvious trauma, including bruising or bleeding.

Complications if left unattended
Eye injuries require immediate medical attention. Failure to seek medical treatment can result in visual impairment, deficit

or permanent loss, particularly if ocular haemorrhaging results following the injury.

Immediate treatment
Cold compress. Avoid pressure on the eye. Seek immediate emergency medical care.

Rehabilitation and prevention
Rehabilitation for an eye injury varies broadly depending on the nature and severity. Minor injuries are generally self-healing, while serious injuries may require ophthalmic surgery and considerable rehabilitation. Eye protection including safety goggles, helmets with eye shields and other eye protection for sports such as cricket, wrestling, football, soccer, hockey, lacrosse, paintball, basketball and racquet sports including tennis should be worn when possible to prevent such injuries.

Long-term prognosis
Prognosis for eye injuries varies according to the nature and severity. Minor injuries that do not damage underlying structures in the eye generally heal given proper attention. More serious injuries, particularly penetrating injuries, run the risk of producing permanent visual loss, and must be treated aggressively as soon after the injury as possible.

EAR

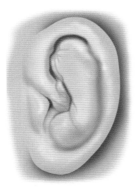

Injuries to the ear can occur when the ear is exposed to direct trauma (from a ball, puck, stick or other object) or through a blow in boxing or as a result of infection, as in the case of swimmer's ear. Cuts and lacerations to the ear are possible in a variety of athletic events,

particularly contact sports, as are bruises and swelling. The eardrum can be ruptured, though this injury in sports is uncommon.

Sports injuries tend to involve the outer or middle ear, rather than the inner ear where the cochlea and other structures reside. For example, cauliflower ear (illustrated) is caused by repeated blunt trauma, where a haematoma forms between the cartilage of the ear and the perichondrium (its fibrous covering).

Cause of injury
Blow to the ear from a ball or other projectile. Sudden pressure change resulting in a ruptured eardrum. Trauma from boxing blow.

Signs and symptoms
Bleeding and swelling. Hearing loss or ringing in the ears. Dizziness and loss of balance.

Complications if left unattended
Ear injuries have potentially serious consequences for long-term hearing and should not be ignored. Ruptured eardrums can also lead to infection, with potentially serious implications.

Immediate treatment
Apply direct pressure should bleeding occur. Sterile cotton in the outer ear to keep the inside of the ear clean.

Rehabilitation and prevention
Cuts and abrasions to the ear as well as cauliflower ear usually heal with minimal medical attention. A ruptured eardrum requires particular care to avoid infection. Ear infections common to swimmers may require antibiotics and usually a period out of the water until the condition is fully resolved. Use of helmets or other headgear in contact sports helps to prevent direct trauma to the ear.

Long-term prognosis
Most athletes experiencing injury to the ear can expect a full recovery, though in the case of a ruptured eardrum partial or in some cases total hearing loss may result. Prompt medical attention is critical for such injuries.

NOSE

Nasal injuries are among the more common sporting injuries, partly due to the protrusion of the nasal bones from the face. Injuries to the nose are generally due to direct blows in contact sports, from cricket balls, basketballs and other athletic equipment or from a fall on the face. In addition to surface cuts, bruising and lacerations to the skin, the nasal bones may be fractured. Blood clotting beneath the mucous membranes of the septum is also possible and is known as a septal haematoma.

Epistaxis, or nosebleed, occurs when superficial blood vessels on the anterior nasal septum are lacerated.

Cause of injury
Blow to the nose from a baseball, basketball or similar object. Blow to the nose from boxing or during contact sports. Fall on the face.

Signs and symptoms
Nasal deformity. Bleeding, pain, or difficulty breathing. Swelling and skin laceration.

Complications if left unattended
Injuries to the nose are potentially dangerous and require prompt medical attention. Collections of clotted blood can accumulate in the space between the nasal cartilage and its fibrous covering, forming a septal haematoma. Resulting pressure on the underlying cartilage can produce irreversible necrosis of the septum. There is also significant risk for infection. If the injury involves damage to the cribriform plate, the athlete can lose cerebrospinal fluid, placing them at risk from meningitis or other serious complications.

Immediate treatment
Apply ice to the nose and elevate the head. Use nasal decongestants to reduce swelling and mucosal congestion.

Rehabilitation and prevention
Most injuries to the nose heal well, though the athlete should avoid contact or other high-risk sports during this phase. Fractures need to be reset but do not in most cases require surgery. Helmets with adequate face protection should be used where the nose is at risk, to help prevent such injuries.

Long-term prognosis
Less serious nasal injuries usually allow the athlete to return to non-contact sports within two weeks. Full healing of fractures usually occurs in three weeks without lasting cosmetic or functional deformity.

REHABILITATION EXERCISES

Lateral neck stretch

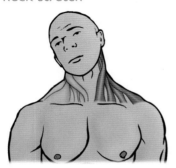

Look forward while keeping your head up. Slowly move your ear toward your shoulder. Keep your hands behind your back and do not lift your shoulder up to your ear.

Neck extension stretch

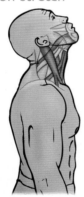

Stand upright and lift your head, looking upward as if trying to point up with your chin. Relax your shoulders and keep your hands by your side.

Forward neck stretch

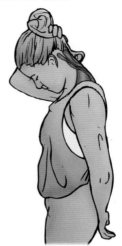

Stand upright and let your chin fall forward toward your chest. Relax your shoulders and keep your hands by your side.

Single arm dumbbell row

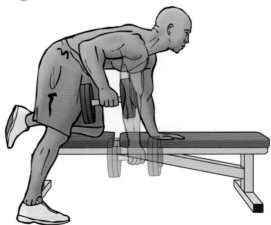

Place your left knee on a weight bench and bend over to rest your left hand on the bench as well. Leaving your other foot on the ground, grip a dumbbell with your right hand. Lift the dumbbell by bending your elbow to a 90-degree angle as if you are starting a lawnmower. Slowly release and repeat.

Isometric lateral neck exercise

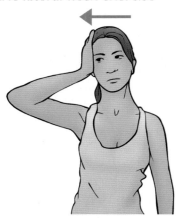

With both feet firmly on the ground, raise one hand and place it above your ear on the side of your head. Push your head gently into your hand until you feel tension in your neck. Release and repeat on the other side of your head.

Isometric rotation neck exercise

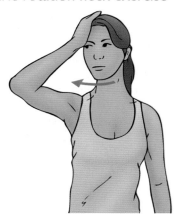

With both feet firmly on the ground, raise one hand and place it slightly forward of your ear. Rotate your head, pushing gently into your hand until you feel tension in your neck. Release and repeat on the other side of your head.

Isometric forward neck exercise

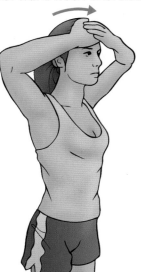

With both feet firmly on the ground, place both hands on your forehead and gently push your head into your hands until you feel tension in the front of your neck.

Isometric rearward neck exercise

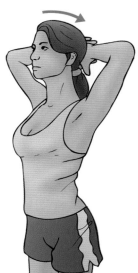

Clench your hands together and place them behind your head. Push your head gently backward into your hands until you feel tension in the back of your neck.

Sports Injuries of the Hand and Fingers

ANATOMY AND PHYSIOLOGY

The five metacarpal bones of the palm run from the carpal bones of the wrist to the base of the fingers. (The knuckles are the heads of the metacarpals where they articulate with the phalanges of the fingers.) Each metacarpal bone comprises a base, shaft, neck and head (from proximal to distal end).

The first metacarpal bone is the shortest and connects with the trapezium at the base of the thumb. The other four metacarpals of the hand connect to the trapezoid, capitate and hamate, and lateral/medial surfaces of the adjoining metacarpals. Each finger has three phalanges, whereas the thumb only has two, making a total of fourteen phalanges.

Each finger of the hand has three joints to enable fine motor control. The metacarpophalangeal (MCP) or knuckle joints are condyloid joints, each of which is enclosed in a capsule that is reinforced by strong collateral ligaments. The carpometacarpal (CMC) joint of the thumb is a saddle joint but the CMC joints of the fingers are plane joints. The intermetacarpal (IM) joints are also plane joints and both the CMC and IM joints are surrounded by a joint capsule. The interphalangeal (IP) joints, both distal (DIP) and proximal (PIP), are hinge joints.

The strong ulnar (medial) collateral ligament of the metacarpophalangeal joint connects the first metacarpal bone to the first phalanx at the base of the thumb. Its function is to prevent the thumb from stretching too far away from the hand. The ligament is required for pinching and grasping activities.

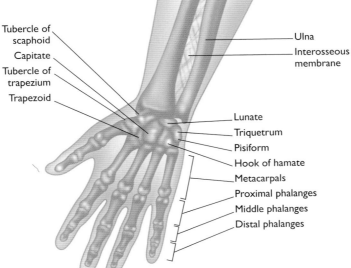

The bones of the right wrist and hand, anterior view.

Extensor tendons are small muscle tendons in the hand and fingers which enable delicate finger movements and hand coordination. They are located on the dorsal aspect of the hand and fingers, allowing the athlete to extend and straighten the fingers and thumb. Extensor tendons attach to muscles in the forearm.

The muscles of the hand can be grouped as: 1) the 'intrinsic' muscles, consisting of the interossei, located between the metacarpals to act on the four fingers and thumb, and the lumbricals, which arise from the tendons of flexor digitorum profundus in the palm and act on the four fingers; 2) the muscles of the hypothenar eminence; 3) the muscles of the thenar eminence; and 4) the adductor pollicis muscle.

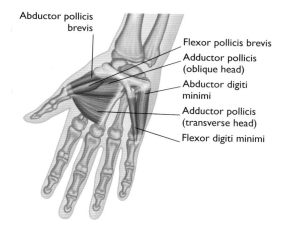
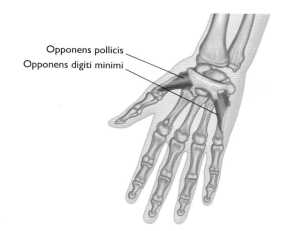

Abductor pollicis brevis

Flexor pollicis brevis
Adductor pollicis (oblique head)
Abductor digiti minimi
Adductor pollicis (transverse head)
Flexor digiti minimi

Opponens pollicis
Opponens digiti minimi

Muscles of the hand.

METACARPAL FRACTURES

Breaks or fractures in one or more of the metacarpal bones may result from a variety of events. They are common in football and basketball players. Metacarpals are vulnerable to direct force and can be fractured when a closed fist strikes another person or hard object, such injuries being referred to as a boxer's fracture. Metacarpal bones can fracture either at the base, shaft or neck. The most common fracture is of the neck of the fifth metacarpal.

Cause of injury
A direct blow to the hand. Falling directly onto the hand. Longitudinal force transmitted through a closed fist when punching.

Signs and symptoms
Local pain and swelling. Bruising and deformity of the broken bone or knuckle. Loss of hand movement and function.

Complications if left unattended
Use of a hand not properly immobilized following metacarpal fracture may lead to lasting deformity and reduced function as well as possible damage to surrounding nerves, muscles, tendons, blood vessels and ligaments.

Immediate treatment
Wash any associated cuts to prevent infection and apply ice to reduce swelling. Elevate the injured hand and avoid using it.

Rehabilitation and prevention
Prevention of metacarpal fractures requires avoidance of activities likely to produce them, particularly striking hard objects with the hand. Preventing further injury to already fractured metacarpals is usually accomplished by immobilizing the hand, either with a finger splint or short cast, depending on the nature of the metacarpal fracture. Exercises designed to gradually increase movement, flexion and extension of the wrist or fingers will help restore full use.

Long-term prognosis
Full recovery from most metacarpal fractures can be expected with aggressive early attention, which may include resetting of the bone and immobilization of the hand. Surgery may be required in the case of displaced bones, with the affected metacarpal realigned and held fast by means of removable pins.

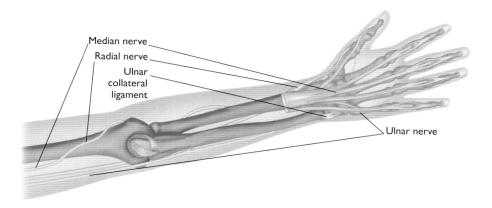

Median nerve
Radial nerve
Ulnar collateral ligament
Ulnar nerve

THUMB SPRAIN

Many activities can pull the thumb suddenly away from the rest of the hand, stretching or occasionally tearing this ligament. The injury is prevalent among skiers and is often referred to as skier's thumb, though repetitive activities that gradually wear and irritate the collateral ligaments, fibrous bands of tissue lying on either side of the thumb, can produce a chronic form of injury.

Cause of injury
Thumb being jammed into another player, piece of equipment or the ground. Repetitive wear of the ulnar collateral ligament through gripping between the thumb and index finger. Any activity that violently separates the thumb from the rest of the hand, such as a skiing fall.

Signs and symptoms
Local pain and swelling over the torn ligament. Difficulty grasping objects or holding them firmly. Instability of the thumb which may repeatedly catch on objects or clothing.

Complications if left unattended
If a torn ulnar collateral ligament is left untreated it may result in a painful, unstable thumb with loss of mobility. Continued soreness and a propensity for re-injury are also possible.

Immediate treatment
Elevate and ice for thirty minutes every two hours. Immobilize with a splint.

Rehabilitation and prevention
Buddy taping the thumb to its neighbouring digit, especially during contact sports, may help prevent re-injury. Gradual use of motion exercises to restore thumb movement should be undertaken as the ulnar collateral ligament undergoes final repair.

Long-term prognosis
Non-contact sports may usually be permitted six weeks following the injury, and a return to contact sports can be expected after three months, depending on the severity of the original sprain.

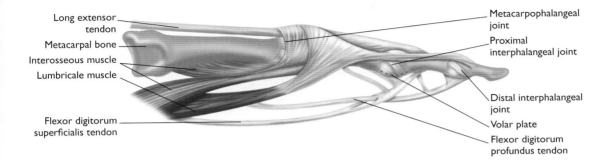

Long extensor tendon
Metacarpal bone
Interosseous muscle
Lumbricale muscle
Flexor digitorum superficialis tendon

Metacarpophalangeal joint
Proximal interphalangeal joint
Distal interphalangeal joint
Volar plate
Flexor digitorum profundus tendon

MALLET FINGER

Extensor tendons are vulnerable to injury, lying just below the skin surface directly on the bones of the back of the hand and fingers. Such tendons may be torn apart when a finger is jammed, separating the tendons from their attachment to bone. The injury is common at the start of the season for sports like baseball, basketball and netball, often caused by a ball hitting the fingertip. When an object hits the fingertip it pushes it sharply down. The forceful flexion avulses the lateral bands of the extensor tendon from its attachment to the phalanx. Cuts to the hand or fingers can also damage the extensor tendons.

Cause of injury

Cuts or lacerations affecting the backs of the fingers and hands. Baseball, volleyball, football, basketball or other object striking the fingertips while the extensor tendon is taut. Jamming the finger against a wall, door or other immovable object.

Signs and symptoms

Inability to straighten the finger. Bruising, pain and swelling of the affected finger. Drooping fingertip.

Complications if left unattended

Left untreated, mallet finger may cause permanent cosmetic deformity in the finger, though often without further complication. Without splinting, some residual stiffness and loss of finger extension may result. Surgical intervention is typically not advised in simple cases of mallet finger as surgical complications may include stiffness, nail bed damage, infection and chronic tenderness.

Immediate treatment

RICER regimen for the first two days, followed by heat treatment. Immobilization with a splint pending medical consultation.

Rehabilitation and prevention

Generally a splint must be worn continuously until the extensor tendon is fully healed. It will often require several months for local swelling and redness to fully subside. Special care with the fingertips should always be taken in sports involving fast-moving balls, as well as when handling cutting implements.

Long-term prognosis

With attention to post-injury care including immobilization of the injured finger, most athletes achieve full restoration of movement and appearance of the digit.

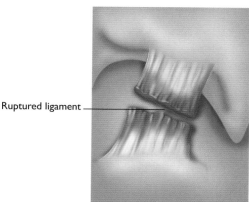

Ruptured ligament

FINGER SPRAIN

Finger sprains are injuries to a joint that cause a stretch or tear in a ligament. These sprains are common in a wide variety of sports including football, basketball, cricket and handball. They include MCP and IP sprains, Boutonnière deformity and mallet finger.

Injuries to the PIP joint (the middle joint of the finger) are most common, and may result when the joint is bent back (hyperextension). This can cause rupture or tearing of the volar plate (see page 89), a ligament connecting the proximal and middle phalanges to the collateral ligaments found on either side of the PIP joint.

Cause of injury
Blow to the hand at the region of the joint. Hyperextension of the joint, damaging the volar plate ligament. Collateral ligaments are overstretched in a side-to-side displacement.

Signs and symptoms
Pain and tenderness in the finger. Pain when moving the finger joint. Swelling of the middle finger joint, with deformity in the case of joint displacement.

Complications if left unattended
Should a deformity associated with finger sprain become chronic, the chances of successful surgical correction are reduced. Potential for permanent functional deficit in the injured finger exists.

Immediate treatment
Use of anti-inflammatory or other pain medication to reduce swelling. Apply ice packs to the injured finger for 20–30 minutes every 3–4 hours for 2–3 days or until pain subsides.

Rehabilitation and prevention
Most finger sprain injuries, depending on severity, will be splinted or buddy taped to neighbouring digits in order to immobilize the area of trauma. Finger strains tend to be unforeseen and unpreventable injuries, though proper sports technique and equipment may reduce the likelihood of some sprains. Strengthening and mobility exercises for the fingers may be undertaken following initial healing.

Long-term prognosis
Full recovery and restoration of function in the injured finger is likely in most cases of finger sprains.

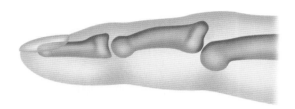

FINGER DISLOCATION

Finger dislocations are more severe injuries than sprains and involve the displacement of the joint, altering the alignment of the finger. The joint must therefore be reset before the finger is immobilized with casting, splint or taping. Splints allow the ligaments and joint capsule to properly heal. Such dislocations are common in many sports, particularly contact sports in which the athlete's hands come into direct physical contact with other players (football, wrestling) and sports emphasizing use of the hands (volleyball, baseball, basketball, gymnastics, karate etc.).

Dislocation of a joint involves the tearing of ligaments and the joint capsule surrounding the affected joint. Dislocation may occur in any of the joints of the fingers. Dislocation of the IP joints occurs most commonly in basketball and football. Dislocations of the MCP and CMC joints can occur during falls onto the outstretched hand.

Cause of injury
Fingers being struck by a football, baseball, basketball, etc. Falling onto the outstretched hand. Abduction force applied to the thumb, as in a skier's fall.

Signs and symptoms
Immediate pain and swelling. Finger appears crooked. Inability to straighten or bend the dislocated joint.

Complications if left unattended
Deformity of the joint, loss of function and early-onset arthritis can accompany an untreated finger dislocation. While some dislocations correct themselves without medical intervention, generally the displaced joint must be reset by a physician, followed by immobilization during the healing of the injury.

Immediate treatment
RICER treatment should immediately follow the injury. Avoid all unnecessary movement of the injured finger.

Rehabilitation and prevention
Ligaments occasionally do not heal adequately following dislocation, and surgery may be required to repair damaged structures. Generally finger dislocations are successfully treated by resetting the misaligned joint and holding the area rigid by means of a splint until thorough healing of the ligament and joint capsule has taken place. Stretching, strengthening and mobility exercises may follow to avoid stiffening or mobility loss in the affected joint.

Long-term prognosis
Most finger dislocations do not result in long-term finger deformity or loss of function, and a full recovery may be expected given aggressive early treatment.

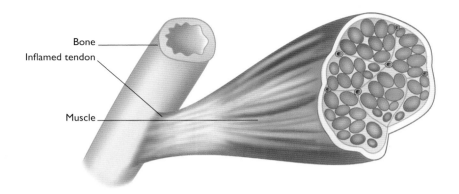

Bone

Inflamed tendon

Muscle

HAND/FINGER TENDINITIS

Tendinitis means irritation and inflammation of tendons and may affect any of the tendons of the wrist or fingers. The affliction is common where overuse or overworking of the tendons is involved but can also be related to various underlying diseases including diabetes and rheumatoid arthritis.

Tendons are resilient cords of tissue connecting muscle to bone, and act to transmit forces between the muscle and the skeleton which requires them to bear considerable mechanical loads. Overworking of the tendons can lead to inflammation of the tendons and their tendon sheaths. Tendinitis may be accompanied by fibrinoid necrosis and myxomatous degeneration (a condition where mucus accumulates in connective tissue).

Cause of injury
Intense or sustained exertion involving the tendons of the wrist or hand. Lack of adequate recovery time between athletic exertion. Cold temperatures or constant vibration in the hand.

Signs and symptoms
Tenderness. Inflammation. Crackling or grating sensation under the skin (crepitus).

Complications if left unattended
Should athletic activity continue despite existing tendinitis, the affliction can become chronic and permanent damage to the structure of the tendons may result.

Immediate treatment
Anti-inflammatory medication. Ice for the first 24–48 hours after onset of the condition.

Rehabilitation and prevention
Following rest and measures to reduce inflammation, strengthening and stretching exercises targeting the affected tendons can be undertaken, provided pain has subsided. Avoidance of repetitive stress to the tendons and ensuring proper recovery time following physical activities involving the wrist and hands can help prevent recurrence of the condition.

Long-term prognosis
Proper care of tendinitis usually results in reduction of inflammation, alleviation of pain and full recovery of movement, though the condition can become chronic, particularly in elite athletes whose schedule demands repeated over-stress of tendons.

REHABILITATION EXERCISES

Finger squashing (flexion)

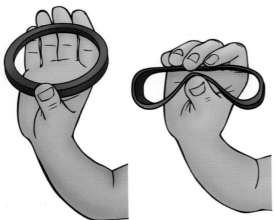

Grip the ring with four fingers on top and your thumb on the bottom. Close your hand so that your thumb meets your middle finger. Repeat.

Finger opening (extension)

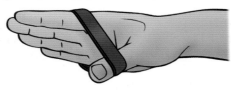

Put your hand inside the ring, but do not push it past your knuckles. Stretch your fingers apart by attempting to get your middle finger and thumb as far away from each other as possible.

Palms-out forearm stretch

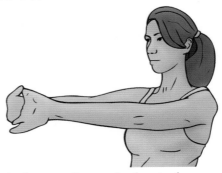

Interlock your fingers in front of your chest and then straighten your arms and turn the palms of your hands outward.

Finger stretch

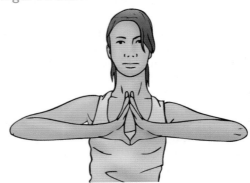

Place the tips of your fingers together and push your palms toward each other.

Thumb stretch

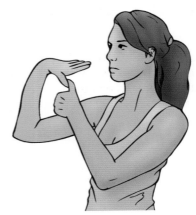

Start with your fingers pointing up and your thumb out to one side, then use your other hand to pull your thumb down.

ANATOMY AND PHYSIOLOGY

The wrist helps orient and support the hand. The wrist can be thought of as a multi-articular complex. Most wrist movement occurs at the radiocarpal joint, an ellipsoid joint. The distal surface of the radius and a fibrocartilage disc articulate with the proximal row of carpal bones: the scaphoid, lunate and triquetrum.

Movements at the radiocarpal joint occur in combination with the midcarpal and intercarpal joints. These are a series of plane joints, with articulations between the two carpal rows – the midcarpal joint – forming a compound saddle joint. There are numerous intercarpal articulations between the bones of the proximal and distal carpal rows. The distal radioulnar joint is immediately adjacent to the radiocarpal joint. A cartilaginous disc separates the distal ulna and radius from the lunate and triquetrum. An elaborate complex of ligaments holds the bones of the wrist together and allows for their proper coordination. Tendons of muscles passing across the wrist are encased in tendon sheaths known as the tenosynovium.

Three major nerves supply the skin and muscles of the forearm, hand and fingers: the median, radial and ulnar nerves. These nerves are vulnerable to injury and compression at several points on their paths.

The carpal tunnel is a narrow, rigid space formed by the shape of the carpal bones and ligaments at the base of the hand. The median nerve and the tendons of the flexor muscles of the hand and fingers run through it. The median nerve is vulnerable to compression in the carpal tunnel. It transmits sensory information from the palmar aspect of the thumb and first two or three fingers as well as supplying some of the muscles of the hand.

The elbow has two bony points frequently associated with ulnar nerve compression (ulnar tunnel syndrome): the olecranon process and the medial epicondyle of the humerus. The space between these bony protrusions is known as the ulnar tunnel and the ulnar nerve passes through it, running down the forearm and into the hand. The ulnar nerve acts on the adductor pollicis muscle which pulls the thumb toward the palm of the hand and controls small intrinsic muscles of the hand. It also transmits sensory information from the medial border of the hand and the fourth and fifth fingers.

The anterior forearm contains three functional muscle groups: the pronators of the forearm; the wrist flexors; and the long flexors of the fingers and thumb. They are arranged in three layers: the superficial layer comprises four muscles: pronator teres, flexor carpi radialis, palmaris longus and flexor carpi ulnaris. The middle layer contains only flexor digitorum superficialis. The deepest layer consists of: flexor digitorum profundus, flexor pollicis longus and pronator quadratus. On the back of the forearm there are two muscle groups. The superficial group contains, from the radial to ulnar side: brachioradialis, extensor carpi radialis longus, extensor carpi radialis brevis, extensor digitorum, extensor digiti minimi and extensor carpi ulnaris. The muscle belly of brachioradialis is prominent when working against resistance. The deep group contains: supinator, abductor pollicis longus, extensor pollicis brevis, extensor pollicis longus and extensor indicis.

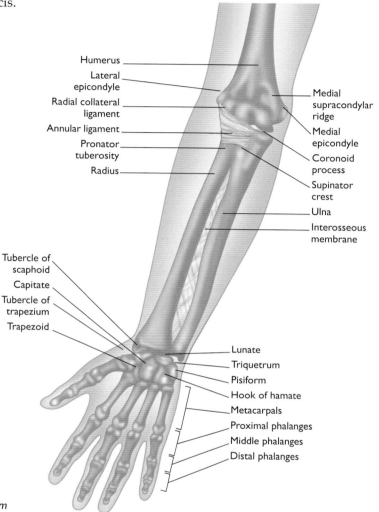

Bones of the right forearm and hand, posterior view.

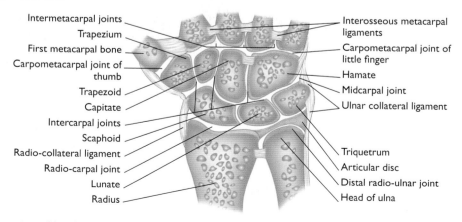

Joints of the wrist and hand, coronal view.

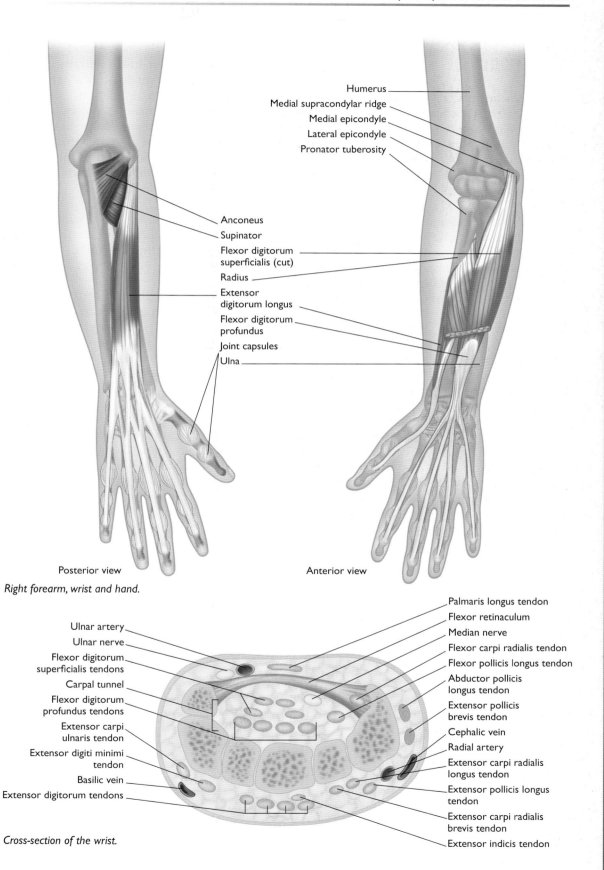

Humerus
Medial supracondylar ridge
Medial epicondyle
Lateral epicondyle
Pronator tuberosity

Anconeus
Supinator
Flexor digitorum
superficialis (cut)
Radius
Extensor
digitorum longus
Flexor digitorum
profundus
Joint capsules
Ulna

Posterior view

Anterior view

Right forearm, wrist and hand.

Ulnar artery
Ulnar nerve
Flexor digitorum
superficialis tendons
Carpal tunnel
Flexor digitorum
profundus tendons
Extensor carpi
ulnaris tendon
Extensor digiti minimi
tendon
Basilic vein
Extensor digitorum tendons

Palmaris longus tendon
Flexor retinaculum
Median nerve
Flexor carpi radialis tendon
Flexor pollicis longus tendon
Abductor pollicis
longus tendon
Extensor pollicis
brevis tendon
Cephalic vein
Radial artery
Extensor carpi radialis
longus tendon
Extensor pollicis longus
tendon
Extensor carpi radialis
brevis tendon
Extensor indicis tendon

Cross-section of the wrist.

WRIST AND FOREARM FRACTURE

Should an athlete fall onto an outstretched wrist, a break or fracture of the wrist or bones of the forearm may result. Sports vulnerable to such injury include running, cycling, skateboarding, rollerblading and other activities in which an outstretched hand may be used to break a fall.

The two most common wrist fractures are Colles' fractures, which occur at the distal end of the radius, and scaphoid fractures, which involve the scaphoid, a small bone that articulates with the radius near the base of the thumb.

Cause of injury
A fall onto an outstretched wrist. A blow to the wrist. Extreme twisting of the wrist.

Signs and symptoms
Deformity of the wrist. Pain and swelling. Limited motion in the thumb or wrist.

Complications if left unattended
Wrist fractures often fuse naturally, though complications may arise in the untreated fracture leading to limitations of wrist movement and forearm pronation and supination. Osteoarthritis may also result from untreated fractures. Untreated or misdiagnosed scaphoid fractures run the risk of non-union or malunion of fractured bone fragments.

Immediate treatment
Apply an ice pack over the wrist to reduce swelling. Elevate the fractured wrist or forearm and place it in a sling.

Rehabilitation and prevention
Immobilization with a rigid cast is generally required for such fractures to properly heal, with X-ray follow-ups to analyze improvement. Where surgery is required, wires or screws may be employed to fuse fractured segments.

Long-term prognosis
Prognosis in the case of radial or ulnar fractures varies. Open fractures (where the skin is broken) tend to have less favorable outcomes. Most scaphoid fractures of the wrist heal thoroughly if immobilized early after injury and allowed to heal for 8–12 weeks.

026:WRIST SPRAIN

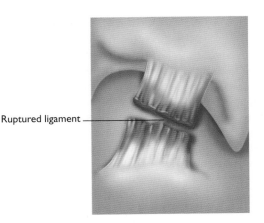

Ruptured ligament

WRIST SPRAIN

Wrist sprains involve injury to the ligaments of the wrist. Such sprains are a common occurrence when the hand is extended to break a fall. Ligaments are necessary for stabilization of the hand and control of motion. Wrist sprains vary from moderate to severe, with the latter involving complete tearing of the ligaments and instability of the associated joint. The injury is common in athletes engaged in football, basketball, skiing, snowboarding, rollerblading and a variety of other sports in which the hands are vulnerable.

The eight carpal bones of the wrist are connected via complex ligaments – fibrous bands of connective tissue. Ligaments also connect the bones of the wrist with the radius and ulna and the metacarpal bones of the hand. The smooth coordination of these bones required for fine hand movement is impaired when one or more ligaments are injured.

Cause of injury
Engaging in sports where falls are common: e.g. in-line skating, snowboarding, cycling, soccer, football, baseball and volleyball. Lack of protective equipment, including wrist guards. Muscle weakness or atrophy.

Signs and symptoms
Pain with movement of the wrist. Burning or tingling feeling at the wrist. Bruising or discolouration of the skin.

Complications if left unattended
Moderate to severe wrist sprains left untreated can lead to ongoing deficit of movement and strength in the wrist as well as developing arthritis at the region of the injury.

Immediate treatment
RICER regimen immediately following injury. Immobilization of injured wrist to restrict movement.

Rehabilitation and prevention
Flexibility and range of motion exercises may be encouraged by a physical therapist, following initial recovery of the ligament. Should the ligament be torn completely, or if fracture accompanies the sprain, surgery may be required. Use of protective guards for wrists and concentration on balance during sport may help to avoid this injury.

Long-term prognosis
Most wrist sprains undergo full recovery given proper initial care and necessary healing time.

WRIST DISLOCATION

Most dislocations of the wrist involve the lunate bone, though other bones may also be involved. When a bone is dislocated, it no longer articulates properly with adjacent bones. The injury affects the soft tissues surrounding the region of dislocation, including muscles, nerves, tendons, ligaments and blood vessels. Dorsal ligaments of the wrist are weaker and more likely to be involved in dislocations.

Cause of injury
Complication of a severe wrist sprain. Hard fall onto an outstretched hand. Congenital abnormality, including malformed joint surfaces.

Signs and symptoms
Loss of hand and wrist movement. Severe pain in the wrist. Numbness or paralysis below the dislocation due to severed blood vessels or nerves.

Complications if left unattended
Outcomes for untreated wrist dislocation are unpredictable. Cases exist of full recovery and restoration of movement. Complications, however, may restrict motion of the wrist and produce ongoing pain, joint stiffness, discomfort and impaired flexibility and movement. Arthritis may also develop in the injured region.

Immediate treatment
Immobilize the wrist and use RICER.

Rehabilitation and prevention
Exercises designed to strengthen wrist muscles and ligaments will help prevent re-injury. Protection of the wrist during athletics, with gloves, wrist guards or taping may also offer some protection against wrist dislocations.

Long-term prognosis
Prognosis depends on the severity of the dislocation and any attendant complications, including fracture. Proper early treatment and appropriate rehabilitation leads to full recovery in most cases.

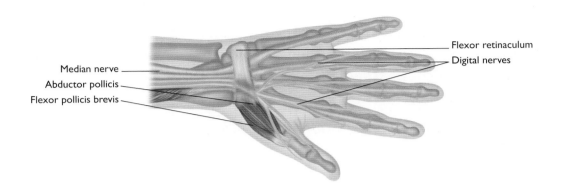

Median nerve

Abductor pollicis

Flexor pollicis brevis

Flexor retinaculum

Digital nerves

CARPAL TUNNEL SYNDROME

Carpal tunnel syndrome (CTS) is a progressive affliction which may be caused by direct trauma or repetitive overuse resulting in compression of the median nerve at the wrist. The condition is three times more likely to affect women, largely due to occupational tasks such as keyboard work. Pregnancy and diabetes are also risk factors.

The carpal tunnel surrounds the median nerve and flexor muscle tendons in their tendon sheaths as they pass from the forearm to the hand. Raised pressure in the tunnel may occur as a result of irritated or inflamed tendons, leading to compression of the median nerve and causing pain, weakness or numbness in the hand which may radiate up the arm. The condition is one of a variety of entrapment neuropathies involving compression or trauma to peripheral nerves.

Cause of injury
Sporting activities that involve repetitive flexion and extension of the wrist, e.g. cycling, throwing events, racket sports and gymnastics. Congenital predisposition. Trauma or injury including fracture or sprain. Occupational tasks.

Signs and symptoms
Burning, numbness or itching in the palm of the hand and fingers. Sensation of finger and wrist swelling. Weakness of grip. Pain that may wake the individual during the night.

Complications if left unattended
Left untreated, CTS can cause loss of sensation in some fingers and permanent weakness of the thumb as the muscles of the thumb atrophy. Heat and cold perception may also be affected in untreated CTS cases.

Immediate treatment
Cease repetitive stress activity causing the condition. Immobilization of the wrist with bandage or splint to prevent further irritation.

Rehabilitation and prevention
Halting the repetitive sport or activity and allowing for rest and rehabilitation time following diagnosis of carpal tunnel syndrome is essential. A bandage or splint may be used to stabilize the injured hand. Releasing the tension in the wrist and hand during sports and periodic exercises to retain mobility and retard stiffness in the hands may help prevent the onset of CTS.

Long-term prognosis
Recurrence of carpal tunnel syndrome following treatment is rare (except in cases of underlying disease such as diabetes). Corticosteroid injections and surgery in persistent cases. The majority of patients properly attending to the injury recover completely.

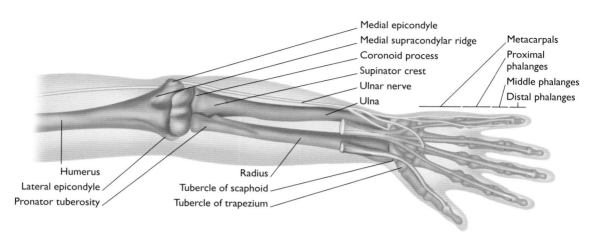

Medial epicondyle
Medial supracondylar ridge
Coronoid process
Supinator crest
Ulnar nerve
Ulna
Metacarpals
Proximal phalanges
Middle phalanges
Distal phalanges
Humerus
Lateral epicondyle
Pronator tuberosity
Radius
Tubercle of scaphoid
Tubercle of trapezium

ULNAR TUNNEL SYNDROME

One of three major nerves responsible for motor function and sensation in the hand, the ulnar nerve runs along the inside of the forearm down to the heel of the hand. In the hand, the ulnar nerve radiates across the palm and into the little finger and ring finger. Pressure on the ulnar nerve can result in pain, loss of sensation and muscle weakness in the hand.

Cause of injury
Overuse of muscles and tendons of the forearm, especially in golf and sports involving throwing. Abnormal growth in the wrist, such as a cyst. Sudden trauma to the ulnar nerve within the ulnar tunnel.

Signs and symptoms
Weakness and increasing numbness on the little finger (medial) side of the hand. Difficulty grasping and holding objects. Tingling along the inner forearm, especially when the elbow is bent.

Complications if left unattended
Without proper treatment, ulnar tunnel syndrome can lead to permanent nerve damage and chronic weakening and numbness due to reduced blood supply to the ulnar nerve.

Immediate treatment
Cease the activity which is causing pressure on the ulnar nerve, and avoid keeping the elbow in a bent position. Splint or pad, especially at night to keep the arm straight.

Rehabilitation and prevention
In the case of ulnar tunnel syndrome due to an abnormal growth such as a cyst, surgery may be required. Where repetitive stress or exercise have led to ulnar nerve inflammation, non-surgical physical therapy including strengthening exercises will often yield improvement in 4–6 weeks. A pad or splint may be used to reduce symptoms at night.

Long-term prognosis
In cases where ulnar tunnel syndrome receives prompt and appropriate attention, the prognosis for full recovery is good. Nerve damage and deficit can result, however, should the condition be allowed to persist without care.

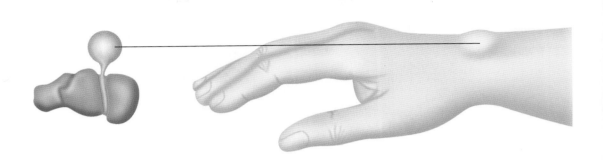

WRIST GANGLION CYST

Ganglion cysts are thin, fibrous capsules containing a clear, mucinous fluid. They feel soft and mobile. Ganglion cysts are connected to an underlying joint capsule or ligament via a thin stalk. They can involve any joint in the hand or wrist but occur mainly on tendon attachments and are palpable between the extensor tendons of the forearm muscles. A ganglion cyst forms when tissue around the joint becomes inflamed and swells with fluid. As this happens, the balloon-like ganglion grows in the connective tissue of the joint or even in the membrane that covers the nearby tendon. Often, cysts are associated with the scapholunate ligament and scaphotrapezial joint of the wrist. Most cysts occur at the dorsal wrist, volar wrist and volar retinacular or distal interphalangeal areas.

Most often, ganglion cysts occur in the 25–45 year-old age group, and are more common in women than in men. Ganglion cysts are benign tumours (so do not spread to other body areas), and their cause is unknown. Sometimes they are also called synovial hernias or synovial cysts because of their relationship to the synovial cavities in the joint. Also known as subchondral cysts.

Cause of injury
Flaw in the joint capsule. Flaw in the tendon sheath. Tissue trauma.

Signs and symptoms
Swollen, sac-like area which changes size. May or may not produce pain. Wrist weakness.

Complications if left unattended
Most ganglion cysts disappear without treatment, though in some cases they recur over time. Such cysts generally do not pose a serious health risk, even if left untreated, though pain and weakness of the wrist may persist without medical care.

Immediate treatment
Ice three times a day if the cyst is painful. Aspirin or anti-inflammatory medication.

Rehabilitation and prevention
Cysts may be drained of fluid by a physician. The patient should not attempt this. Often, cysts will gradually disappear without draining or surgical intervention though they may recur. If the ganglion cyst is painful, sports involving intensive use of the wrist should be limited or avoided until shrinkage or disappearance of the cyst.

Long-term prognosis
Cysts may be asymptomatic and self-limiting. Should medical attention be required the prognosis for full recovery is excellent.

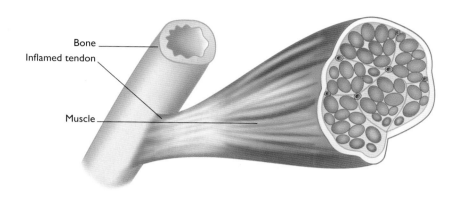

Bone

Inflamed tendon

Muscle

WRIST TENDINITIS

Wrist tendinitis is caused by irritation and inflammation of one or more tendons around the wrist joint. Wrist tendinitis tends to occur in areas where the tendons cross each other or pass over an underlying bony structure, and affects individuals involved in strenuous and repetitive training.

The tendons of the wrist are encased in tendon sheaths known as the tenosynovium. Such sheaths provide for the smooth, friction-free sliding of tendons in the wrist. Swelling, irritation and inflammation of the tenosynovium causes a thickening of the sheath, which constricts proper movement of the tendons resulting in pain and a related affliction, tenosynovitis. Most wrist tendinitis occurs where a tendon passes through constricted tunnels of fascia.

Four common sites of tendinitis are: the first dorsal compartment affecting the abductor pollicis longus and extensor pollicis brevis muscles of the thumb (De Quervain's tenosynovitis); the digital flexor muscles (trigger finger); flexor carpi radialis tendinitis; and lateral epicondylitis ('tennis elbow').

Cause of injury
Sports involving wrist overuse, including all ball sports, racquet sports, rowing, weightlifting and gymnastics. Repetitive stress from typing or lifting.

Signs and symptoms
Pain in the wrist, particularly at the joint. Inflammation in the region of the affected tendon(s). Limited mobility in the affected wrist.

Complications if left unattended
If the activity causing tendinitis is continued and the condition left untreated, the inflammation and associated pain can worsen. The condition can also lead to permanent weakening of the tendon(s).

Immediate treatment
Immobilize the wrist and use RICER. Anti-inflammatory medication.

Rehabilitation and prevention
Often, a physician will use a splint or brace to prevent movement of the injured wrist. In athletic events tendinitis sometimes results from improper technique. The best therapy for tendinitis is to restrict or temporarily discontinue the activity causing tendon inflammation.

Long-term prognosis
Most enjoy a full recovery from tendinitis, providing the afflicted wrist is permitted proper recuperation from inflammation.

REHABILITATION EXERCISES

Wrist curls

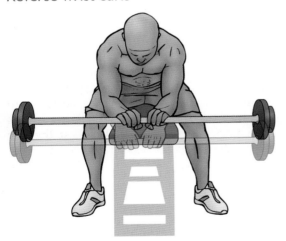

As you sit on a weight bench, bend over slightly at the waist with your elbows resting on your knees. Grip a bench press bar with your palms facing upward. Relax your arms and let the bar inch toward the floor. Flex your wrists upward, without moving your elbows from your knees, then lower the bar.

Reverse wrist curls

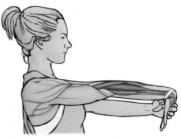

As you sit on a weight bench, bend over slightly at the waist with your elbows resting on your knees. Grip a bench press bar with your palms facing downward. Relax your arms and let the bar inch toward the floor. Extend your wrists upward, without moving your elbows from your knees, then lower the bar.

Plate pinch

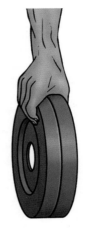

Grip at least two plates in one hand with your thumb on one side and your other fingers on the other. Pinch your thumb and fingers together as tightly as you can.

Wrist stretch

Hold on to your fingers while you straighten your arm. Pull your fingers toward your body.

Rope winding

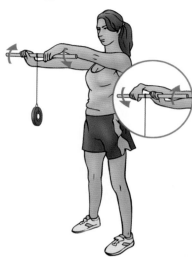

Start with the weight fully unravelled from the bar. Grip the bar with both of your palms facing the floor. Roll the weight up by twisting the bar, then roll the weight down by twisting the bar in the opposite direction.

Rotating wrist stretch

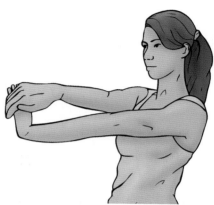

Place one arm straight out in front and parallel to the ground. Rotate your wrist down and outward and then use your other hand to further rotate your hand upward.

Palms-out forearm stretch

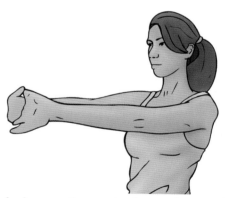

Interlock your fingers in front of your chest and then straighten your arms and turn the palms of your hands outward.

8 Sports Injuries of the Elbow

ANATOMY AND PHYSIOLOGY

The elbow is a hinge joint comprised of three bones: the humerus of the upper arm and the two bones of the forearm – the ulna and the radius. The elbow encompasses three articulations – the humeroulnar, humeroradial and proximal radioulnar joints. Of the forearm bones the ulna is the most medial, being on the little finger side, and is also the largest. At the distal end of the humerus are the trochlea and the capitulum, bony features that articulate with the radius and ulna.

The elbow is reinforced by several important ligaments, the two most important being the ulnar (medial) collateral ligament and the radial (lateral) collateral ligament. The medial collateral ligament is composed of three strong bands that reinforce the medial side of the joint capsule. The lateral collateral ligament is a strong triangular ligament that reinforces the lateral side of the capsule. These ligaments connect the humerus to the ulna and act together to stabilize the elbow. Additionally, the annular ligament envelopes the head of the radius and holds it firmly against the ulna to form the proximal radioulnar joint.

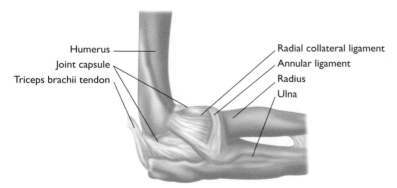

Humerus
Joint capsule
Triceps brachii tendon

Radial collateral ligament
Annular ligament
Radius
Ulna

The elbow joint, right arm, lateral view.

The elbow allows flexion and extension capacity as well as the ability to pronate and supinate, affording a great range of motion. Considerable force is required to dislocate the elbow joint.

The bony prominence at the tip of the elbow is known as the olecranon process of the ulna. The fluid-filled sac located at the olecranon process is the olecranon bursa. It is the largest bursa in the elbow region and provides cushioning protection to the underlying bone.

The lateral epicondyle of the humerus is an important bony feature located just proximal to the outside of the elbow joint. Many muscles attach to the lateral epicondyle, including the common tendon of the forearm extensor muscles, anconeus and the supinator muscle, which is involved in supination (rotating the forearm to the palm up position).

The medial epicondyle is a bony prominence on the inside of the elbow. It is the insertion point for the muscles used to flex the wrist and fingers and for pronation (rotating the forearm to the palm down position).

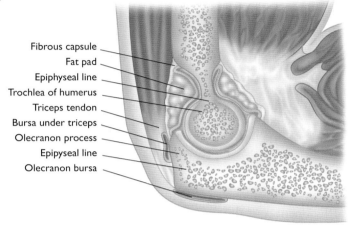

Fibrous capsule
Fat pad
Epiphyseal line
Trochlea of humerus
Triceps tendon
Bursa under triceps
Olecranon process
Epipyseal line
Olecranon bursa

The elbow joint, right arm, mid-sagittal view.

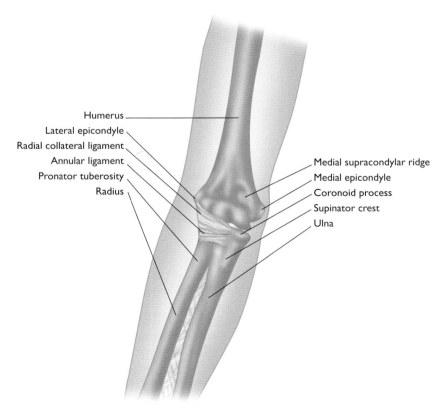

Humerus
Lateral epicondyle
Radial collateral ligament
Annular ligament
Pronator tuberosity
Radius

Medial supracondylar ridge
Medial epicondyle
Coronoid process
Supinator crest
Ulna

The elbow joint, anterior view.

The muscles of the arm originate from the scapula and/or the humerus and insert onto the radius and/or ulna to act upon the elbow joint. They are: biceps brachii; brachialis; triceps brachii and anconeus. (Coracobrachialis, although acting upon the shoulder joint, is also included because of its proximity to the other muscles of this group.) Biceps brachii is the main supinator of the forearm and has two tendinous heads at its origin and two tendinous insertions. The short head of biceps forms part of the lateral wall of the axilla along with coracobrachialis and the humerus. Brachialis lies posterior to biceps brachii and is the main flexor of the elbow joint. Triceps brachii originates from three heads and is the only muscle on the back of the arm. The triceps brachii tendon permits the elbow to straighten with force during certain activities, e.g. push-ups. The tendon of triceps begins around the middle of the muscle and consists of two segments, one covering the back of the lower half of the muscle, the other more deeply situated within the muscle. The two segments or lamellæ join each other above the elbow and insert onto the olecranon.

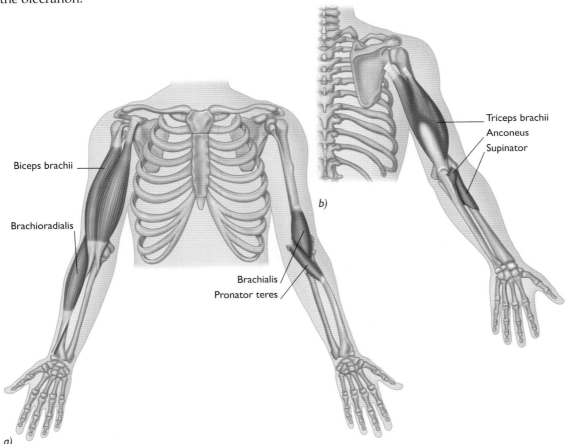

Elbow joint muscles; a) anterior view, b) posterior view.

ELBOW FRACTURE

An elbow fracture is a break involving any of the three arm bones that work together to form the elbow joint. Such fractures may occur as the result of a blunt force striking the elbow during athletics or from a fall onto the elbow. The injury is common to many sports, particularly contact sports such as football. Fractures may be classified as distal humeral fractures, radial fractures and ulnar fractures. Fractures of the radial head are the most common.

Cause of injury
Falling directly onto the elbow. Direct trauma to the elbow. Severe torsion of the elbow beyond its normal range of motion.

Signs and symptoms
Swelling and pain in the region of the elbow. Deformity of the elbow due to bone fracture. Loss of arm mobility.

Complications if left unattended
Without treatment, fractured bones of the elbow can fail to heal properly, and at times fuse in misalignment. This can lead to long-term deficit in range of motion and strength, increased vulnerability to re-injury and deformity of the joint.

Immediate treatment
Apply ice immediately to the swollen area. Immobilize the arm in a splint or sling before seeking emergency help.

Rehabilitation and prevention
Elbow fractures occur from sudden, accidental trauma and are often difficult to prevent. Avoiding athletics at periods of extreme fatigue and protection of the elbow with padding during athletics are both prudent. Additionally, consuming calcium and performing bone strengthening exercises may help avoid fractures.

Long-term prognosis
Long-term prospects for elbow fractures vary depending on the nature and severity of the fracture as well as the age and medical history of the injured athlete. Infections, stiffening of the elbow joint, arthritis, non-union or malunion of bone are possible. In the case of less severe elbow fractures, full recovery may be expected, though the healing process often requires several months.

ELBOW SPRAIN

Ligaments are strong bands of tissue connecting bones and act to stabilize the elbow. A sprain involves the stretching or tearing of elbow ligaments. Many sports are prone to elbow sprains, particularly sports involving throwing, and often involve the medial collateral ligament. Elbow sprains are also common in gymnastics.

Cause of injury
Sudden, abnormal twisting of the arm. Falling onto an outstretched arm. Deficient strength in arm ligaments and muscles.

Signs and symptoms
Pain, tenderness and swelling in the area of the elbow joint. Bruising around the elbow. Limited range of motion in the arm.

Complications if left unattended
Sprains, particularly when they are severe, can lead to future painful or disabling symptoms, including instability and weakness in the elbow, limited range of motion and osteoarthritis.

Immediate treatment
RICER regimen to reduce inflammation and treat pain. Immobilization of injured elbow with a sling or splint.

Rehabilitation and prevention
Proper athletic technique, avoiding exercise during periods of fatigue and protective sportswear including padding can all reduce the risk of elbow sprains. Following initial healing, range of motion exercises and gradual return to athletic activity will help restore flexibility. For a time a supportive brace may be used to prevent sudden re-injury.

Long-term prognosis
Depending on the severity of the sprain and general health of the patient, minor sprains heal thoroughly without future complication. Older athletes or those who have suffered severe sprain (including sprains occurring in conjunction with fractures or dislocations) may suffer some impairment of movement and pain associated with arthritis.

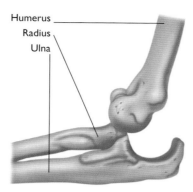

Humerus
Radius
Ulna

(a) Elbow dislocation.

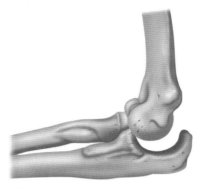

(b) Elbow subluxation.

ELBOW DISLOCATION

Dislocation of the elbow occurs when the humerus is separated by force from where it articulates with the ulna and/or radius. The injury typically produces considerable pain, swellings and loss of movement in the injured arm. Contact sports are more prone to such injuries. Fractures as well as injuries to arteries and nerves sometimes accompany dislocation. A partial dislocation is known as a subluxation.

Cause of injury
Blow or other trauma to the elbow. Fall onto an outstretched arm. Violent contact between the elbow and another athlete or object.

Signs and symptoms
Severe pain in the elbow, swelling and bruising. Loss of range of motion. Loss of feeling in the hand following sharp injury to the elbow.

Complications if left unattended
Improper healing can follow if a dislocation is left untreated, causing nerve and arterial damage, osteoarthritis, ongoing pain in the injured arm, loss of full movement and distortion of the elbow joint. Infection of the dislocated region is also possible, particularly if a fracture is involved.

Immediate treatment
Check for possible damage to an artery by taking the pulse. Treat the injury with ice and immobilize the elbow in a splint or sling.

Rehabilitation and prevention
Ice should be used to reduce initial pain and swelling, while proper medical attention is sought. The elbow should be moved as little as possible and elevated frequently. Proper attention to athletic technique and padding of the elbow region, especially in the case of contact sports such as football, may help prevent such injuries.

Long-term prognosis
Generally, dislocations without further complications of nerve or arterial damage heal thoroughly given proper initial care and some rehabilitative exercises.

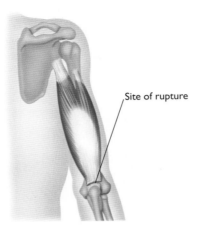

Site of rupture

TRICEPS BRACHII TENDON RUPTURE

The triceps brachii tendon is located at the back of the upper arm, inserting onto the back of the elbow. A direct fall onto an outstretched hand can rupture this tendon (tendon avulsion) though the injury is fairly uncommon. Weightlifters and football linemen are among the athletes who run a risk of triceps brachii tendon rupture due to excessive weight on the tendon.

Cause of injury
Fall onto an outstretched hand, with the elbow in mid-flexion. Excessive weightlifting. Underlying health issues such as diabetes mellitus. It is believed the use of anabolic steroids increases the risk of tendon rupture.

Signs and symptoms
Pain and swelling at the back of the elbow. Inability to straighten the elbow. Muscle spasm.

Complications if left unattended
The injury generally requires surgery to repair. Failure to repair a ruptured triceps brachii tendon can cause permanent tendon deficiency, leading to muscle weakness, continued pain loss of elbow mobility and weightbearing capacity.

Immediate treatment
RICER regimen to reduce inflammation and treat pain. Prevent movement by immobilizing the injury with a splint or sling.

Rehabilitation and prevention
Following surgery to repair a ruptured triceps brachii tendon, exercises may be used to gradually increase the range of motion, flexibility and strength of the injured arm. Proper technique, particularly if weightlifting or bodybuilding is critical to prevent such injuries.

Long-term prognosis
With surgery soon after the time of injury and proper rehabilitation, ruptures of the triceps brachii tendon generally heal completely, though complications such as accompanying fractures will affect long-term prognosis.

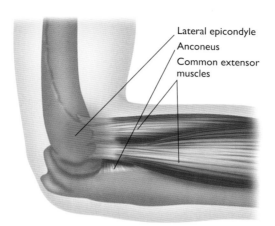

Lateral epicondyle
Anconeus
Common extensor
muscles

TENNIS ELBOW

Tennis elbow, also known as lateral
epicondylitis, is the most common overuse
injury in the adult elbow, and causes the
bony prominence on the outside of the elbow
to become painful and tender. The affliction
is usually related to strain or overuse of the
muscles attaching to the lateral epicondyle of
the humerus or, less frequently, direct trauma
to the elbow.

The extensor muscles of the forearm, which
extend (straighten) the wrist, become strained
from overuse, causing inflammation and pain
where they attach to the bone. The supinator
muscle which allows the forearm to be
twisted to the palm up position also attaches
to the lateral epicondyle and can cause tennis
elbow. Tendons attached to the bones of the
elbow can become restricted or taut, causing
irritation.

Cause of injury
Overuse of the muscles attached to the
elbow. Direct injury to the elbow. Arthritis,
rheumatism or gout.

Signs and symptoms
Outer part of the elbow is painful and tender
to touch. Movement is painful. Elbow is
inflamed.

Complications if left unattended
Tennis elbow is generally treated without
surgery, though discomfort will often worsen,
with the potential for tendon or muscle
damage should the condition be ignored.

Immediate treatment
Avoidance of the activities causing repetitive
stress to the elbow. RICER regimen for
48–72 hours following injury. Use of anti-
inflammatory drugs and analgesics.

Rehabilitation and prevention
Often a splint or bandage will be used to
immobilize the injured elbow and prevent
excess movement. Activities involving
repetitive stress to the elbow or extensor
muscles of the wrist should be avoided until
the condition improves. Should surgery be
required a rest period of six weeks is advised
before strengthening exercises begin.

Long-term prognosis
Few patients suffering from tennis elbow
require surgery. Of the small percentage
that do, 80–90% find the condition markedly
improved.

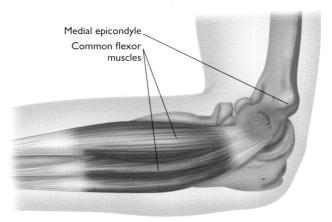

Medial epicondyle
Common flexor
muscles

GOLFER'S ELBOW

Golfer's elbow, also known as medial epicondylitis, is a form of tendinitis similar to tennis elbow. Golfing is one of many sources of the affliction, which can result from any activity leading to overuse of the muscles and tendons of the forearm. While the painful sensation at the elbow is similar to tennis elbow, in the case of golfer's elbow the pain and inflammation occur at the inside (or medial side) of the joint.

The medial epicondyle is a bony prominence on the inside of the elbow. It is the insertion point for muscles used to bend the wrist downward. Forceful, repetitive bending of the fingers and wrist can lead to small ruptures of muscle and tendon in this area. While the golfing swing produces a tightening in the flexor muscles and tendons that can lead to medial epicondylitis, other activities can produce the same injury.

Cause of injury
Sudden trauma or blow to the elbow. Repetitive stress to the flexor muscles and tendons of the forearm. Repeated stress placed on the arm during the acceleration phase of the throwing motion. Underlying health issues including neck problems, rheumatism, arthritis or gout.

Signs and symptoms
Tenderness and pain at the medial epicondyle, which worsens when the wrist is flexed. Pain resulting from lifting or grasping objects. Difficulty extending the forearm.

Complications if left unattended
Golfer's elbow, while generally alleviated by proper rest, can cause increasing pain and unpleasantness if the stressful activity continues. The condition rarely requires surgery and responds well to proper rehabilitation. Should surgery be required, scar tissue is removed from the elbow where the tendons attach.

Immediate treatment
Avoidance of the activities causing repetitive stress to the elbow. RICER regimen for 48–72 hours following the injury. Use of anti-inflammatory drugs and analgesics.

Rehabilitation and prevention
In the case of golfing, the affliction can be reduced in severity or prevented altogether through attention to proper technique and attention to overuse. Golfer's elbow is more prevalent early in the golf season, when muscles and tendons are not yet sufficiently conditioned. Rehabilitation generally involves avoiding the painful activity for a period. Use of analgesics for pain and anti-inflammatory drugs help reduce symptoms. After healing, resistive exercises may be undertaken to improve strength.

Long-term prognosis
Those suffering from golfer's elbow generally make a full recovery without surgery or advanced medical care, provided the injured elbow is afforded proper rest from the stressful activity.

THROWER'S ELBOW

Athletes involved in throwing sports are vulnerable to this condition, which is a result of severe stress to the elbow. The baseball pitch is a common source of thrower's elbow, as well as tennis, volleyball, javelin throwing and cricket. Forceful throwing motions can damage the bones as well as the associated muscles, tendons and ligaments of the elbow. Throwing activity results in a compression of structures on the lateral or outside of the elbow, while simultaneously stretching structures on the medial or inside of the elbow. Lateral compression can cause tiny fractures in the bones of the elbow leading to bone spurs and chips. Medial stretching can cause a painful and debilitating strain to ligaments.

Cause of injury
Repetitive strain from throwing activity. Direct injury to the elbow. Improper athletic technique.

Signs and symptoms
Pain over both sides of the elbow. Weakness, stiffness or numbness of the elbow. Restricted mobility of the forearm due to elbow injury.

Complications if left unattended
Thrower's elbow eventually restricts movement in the arm and causes ongoing pain and inflammation. Bone spurs and chips, calcium formation and the production of scar tissue are all symptomatic of this injury over time if left unattended. Without proper treatment and rehabilitation, pressure on nerves and muscles due to inflammation can restrict blood flow and compress nerves used to control forearm muscles.

Immediate treatment
Avoidance of the activities causing repetitive stress to the elbow. RICER regimen for 48–72 hours following injury. Use of anti-inflammatory drugs and analgesics.

Rehabilitation and prevention
Proper warm-up in order to prepare muscles and tendons for throwing activities is an essential preventive measure. Stretching exercises to maintain suppleness and flexibility of tendons should be an ongoing part of athletic preparation. Bracing and strapping the arm prior to throwing activity may also help to prevent thrower's elbow. Attention to proper equipment and technique is critical. Following a period of recovery from injury, exercises directed at regaining flexibility, endurance and power should be undertaken.

Long-term prognosis
With proper rehabilitation, those suffering from thrower's elbow can generally expect a full recovery, though allowing the problem to worsen can lead to permanent, potentially career-ending restrictions of movement for athletes.

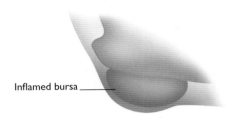

Inflamed bursa

ELBOW BURSITIS

Elbow bursitis, also known as olecranon bursitis, refers to inflammation and swelling of the olecranon bursa. Bursae are small, fluid-filled sacs. They provide gliding or cushioning surfaces that lubricate and reduce friction. Bursae tend to be located adjacent to tendons of major joints, including the shoulders, hips, knees and elbows. Elbow bursitis occurs when the bursa below the tip of the elbow becomes inflamed from leaning on it too much or is injured through direct trauma.

Bursae are typically not visible unless bursitis has caused them to swell and become apparent. Non-inflammatory bursitis usually results from repeated trauma, such as leaning on the elbows, while inflammatory bursitis is the result of infection or an underlying inflammatory medical condition such as rheumatoid arthritis.

Cause of injury
A hard blow to the tip of the elbow, causing the bursa to swell with excess fluid. Leaning on the elbow tip for extended periods. An injury that breaks the skin, causing infection of the bursa.

Signs and symptoms
Pain in the elbow region at rest and during exercise. A rapid and painful swelling on the back of the elbow (red and warm if infected). Swelling may stem from bleeding or seepage of fluid into the bursal sac. Reduced mobility of the elbow.

Complications if left unattended
In addition to continued pain, discomfort and loss of elbow mobility, untreated bursitis can lead to more serious complications, especially when infection is present. In such cases the fluid of the bursa can turn to pus and the infection can intensify and spread in a condition known as septic bursitis, requiring aggressive medical treatment (including antibiotics and occasionally surgical removal of the infected bursa).

Immediate treatment
Rest the afflicted elbow, avoiding all unnecessary pressure. Ice compresses, anti-inflammatory medication and analgesics.

Rehabilitation and prevention
Aspiration by needle to drain fluid and reduce swelling may be needed. Cortisone injections may also be given, which can help prevent re-accumulation of fluid. Barring serious infection, these steps are generally sufficient to treat elbow bursitis. Protecting the elbow during athletics with bracing or padding, and avoiding excessive leaning on the point of the elbow can help prevent the injury.

Long-term prognosis
The long-term outlook for elbow bursitis is generally good, depending on the severity and nature of the injury. Most patients can expect a full recovery, though complications can arise if infection is present, particularly if the condition is not given prompt medical attention.

REHABILITATION EXERCISES

Dumbbell curls

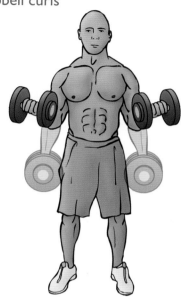

Stand with your feet shoulder width apart and a dumbbell in each hand. Begin by letting the dumbbells rest naturally at your sides. Turn the dumbbells so your palms are facing the ceiling as you bend your elbows and lift the dumbbells up to your chest.

Close grip bench press

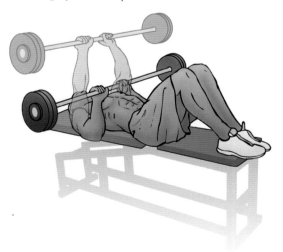

Lie on a weight bench and let the bar relax against your chest with your elbows at your side. Move your hands as close together as possible and lift the bar directly upwards.

Rope press down

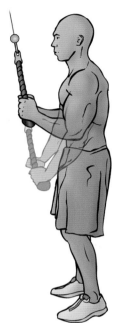

With your feet firmly on the ground, grip a rope with your elbows bent at a 90-degree angle. Pull the rope down by straightening your elbows and bringing your hands toward the floor.

Dumbbell kickbacks

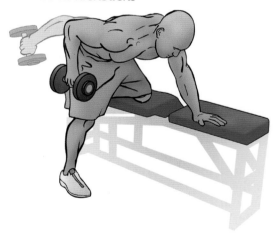

Rest one hand and the same knee on a weight bench. Begin by holding a dumbbell with your elbow at a 90-degree angle in the other hand. Straighten your elbow and push the dumbbell as far behind you as you can. Return to the starting position slowly without letting the dumbbell fall.

Dumbbell overhead extension

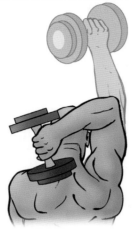

Hold a dumbbell in one hand and put it behind your head letting it fall toward the floor. With your elbow pointing toward the ceiling, raise the dumbbell as high as you can until your elbow is straight. Slowly bring the dumbbell back to the starting position and repeat.

Overhead triceps stretch

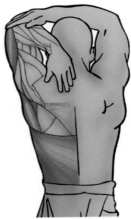

Stand with your hand behind your neck and your elbow pointing upwards. Then use your other hand to pull your elbow down.

Broomstick rotator stretch

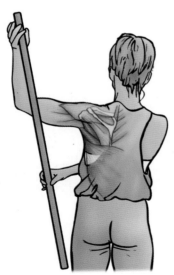

Stand with your arm out and your forearm pointing upwards at 90 degrees. Place a broomstick in your hand and behind your elbow. With your other hand pull the bottom of the broomstick forward.

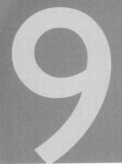

Sports Injuries of the Shoulder and Upper Arm

ANATOMY AND PHYSIOLOGY

The shoulder region is actually composed of three articulations: the sternoclavicular (SC) joint, the acromioclavicular (AC) joint and the glenohumeral (GH) joint. The scapulothoracic articulation describes the movement of the shoulder blade on the chest wall. The articulation referred to specifically as the shoulder joint is the GH joint: the others are joints of the shoulder (or pectoral) girdle. The structure of the shoulder permits a wide arrange of motion, allowing the positioning of the arm and hand.

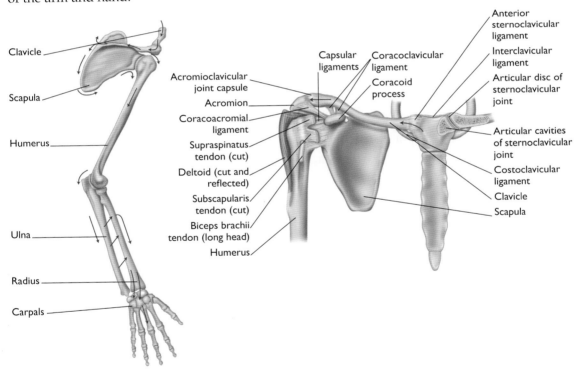

The shoulder region.

The GH joint consists of a ball (formed by the humeral head) and socket (the glenoid cavity). While the GH joint is one of the body's most mobile joints, it is inherently unstable due to the glenoid cavity being only approximately one-third the size of the humeral head (although it is slightly deepened by a rim of fibrocartilage called the glenoid labrum). The GH joint is stabilized by the joint capsule, the glenohumeral, coracohumeral and transverse ligaments, the glenoid labrum and by the rotator cuff muscles.

The clavicle (collarbone) is a slender, curved bone. It acts as a strut attaching the shoulder to the body and works with the scapula to increase range of motion at the shoulder. The clavicle attaches to the sternum medially (the SC joint) and to the acromion process of the scapula laterally (the AC joint). The AC joint is a plane joint. A fibrocartilage articular disc partially divides the articular cavity and absorbs forces and compression. The AC joint is stabilized by the anterior deltoid muscle, the trapezius muscle and by strong stabilizing ligaments.

The SC joint is functionally a ball-and-socket joint but, unlike most articular surfaces, the articular cartilage is fibrocartilage rather than hyaline cartilage. The SC joint is surrounded by a joint capsule, thickened anteriorly and posteriorly by strong stabilizing ligaments. The sternoclavicular joint is strong and generally resistant to dislocation. It has a wide range of movement.

The biceps brachii muscle is located on the front of the upper arm. Its main function is to allow elbow flexion and supination and to support loads placed on the arm. The long and short heads of the muscle have separate points of origin on the scapula and attach via a tendon to the radius and via an aponeurosis to the fascia of the forearm. The tendon of the long head of biceps is closely associated with movements of the GH joint.

The rotator cuff of the shoulder is composed of four muscles: subscapularis, supraspinatus, infraspinatus and teres minor. They help to stabilize the GH joint during movement by keeping the head of the humerus in the glenoid fossa. The subacromial bursa (a fluid-filled sac) is the largest and most commonly injured bursa in the shoulder region. It protects the supraspinatus tendon in the subacromial space where it is prone to impingement.

Along with the pectoralis minor, the large pectoralis major muscle forms the anterior wall of the axilla. It has a wide origin in the clavicle, sternum and first six costal cartilages and inserts on the bicipital groove of the humerus. Pectoralis major adducts and medially rotates the arm at the shoulder. The clavicular portion allows the humerus to be brought up to the horizontal and the direction of the sternocostal fibres allows the arm to be extended against resistance, for example, when doing press-ups. It is an important muscle in climbing, throwing and punching.

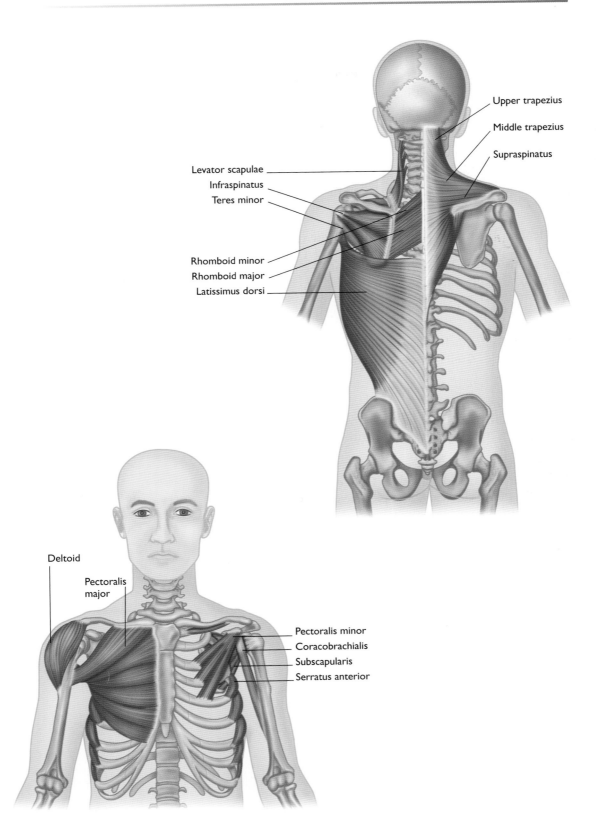

Shoulder girdle muscles.

FRACTURE (COLLARBONE, HUMERUS)

Fractures of the shoulder usually involve a break in either the clavicle, the neck of the humerus or both. Impact injuries involving a sudden blow to the shoulder or a fall are usually responsible. Contact sports including football and rugby can result in shoulder fractures following a violent collision of two players.

Clavicular fractures are common, often resulting from a fall onto the lateral shoulder or an outstretched arm. Fractures of the humerus are generally the result of a fall on an outstretched arm.

Cause of injury
Fall on an outstretched arm. Sudden blow to the clavicle. Collision of two athletes in sports.

Signs and symptoms
Severe pain. Redness and bruising around the site of injury. Inability to raise the arm.

Complications if left unattended
Complications are uncommon. Due to the proximity of the clavicle to the pleurae of the lungs and underlying nerve and blood vessels, pneumothorax, haemothorax and injury to the brachial plexus or subclavian vessels are possible, requiring medical intervention. Chronic pain, decreased range of motion and stiffness due to osteoarthritis may result should the injury be given insufficient time to heal.

Immediate treatment
Ice and analgesics for pain. Immobilization of the injured arm with a sling.

Rehabilitation and prevention
Bones of the clavicle and humerus must be realigned following fracture so that proper healing may ensue. Healing occurs while the clavicle and arm bones are held in place with a strap or sling. After healing, physical therapy including range of motion and strengthening exercises should be undertaken to restore full movement and flexibility.

Long-term prognosis
Most shoulder fractures are successfully treated without resort to surgery, although this is occasionally required for fractures of the clavicle. For less severe fractures, full recovery and restoration of mobility may be expected. In the case of more severe fractures and particularly in older patients, some loss of motion and the possibility of osteoarthritis exist.

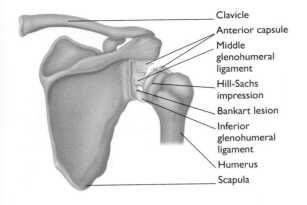

Clavicle
Anterior capsule
Middle glenohumeral ligament
Hill-Sachs impression
Bankart lesion
Inferior glenohumeral ligament
Humerus
Scapula

DISLOCATION OF THE SHOULDER

Dislocation of the shoulder at the GH joint may occur when an athlete falls on an outstretched hand or during abduction and external rotation of the shoulder. Significant force is required to dislocate a shoulder unless the athlete is experiencing re-injury. A shoulder dislocation occurs when the head of the humerus pulls free of the glenoid fossa of the scapula.

While several types of shoulder dislocation exist, the most common is anterior dislocation which represents 95% of all cases. In this dislocation injury, the structures responsible for stabilizing the anterior shoulder, including the capsule and the inferior glenohumeral ligament, are torn free from the bone. Compression fractures of the posteromedial humeral head known as Hill-Sachs lesions are associated with anterior dislocations. More commonly, avulsion of the anterior glenoid labrum can occur, which is known as a Bankart lesion.

Cause of injury
Violent contact with another athlete or solid object. A fall onto an outstretched hand. Sudden, violent torsion of the shoulder.

Signs and symptoms
Severe pain in the shoulder. Arm held away from the body at the side, with the forearm turned outward. Irregular contour of the deltoid muscles.

Complications if left unattended
Dislocation of the GH joint causes damage to the joint ligaments, resulting in the joint becoming less stable and considerably more prone to successive dislocations during athletics. Immobilization of the shoulder during the healing phase does not fully prevent such re-injury, which may require surgical intervention, since the immobilized ligaments often fail to heal in the proper position. Damage to the axillary artery and nerve can also occur, causing weakness in the deltoid muscle.

Immediate treatment
Realignment or reduction of the dislocated joint. Immobilization and analgesics for pain.

Rehabilitation and prevention
Most initial shoulder dislocations are treated without resort to surgery, although subsequent dislocations may require surgical care. Many athletes suffer a range of disabilities following dislocation. An alternative to surgical treatment – prolotherapy – involves injections directed at the anterior shoulder capsule and the insertions of the middle and inferior glenohumeral ligaments. This may offer better relief from pain, restoration of mobility and a speedier return to athletic activity. Further, the technique avoids the formation of scar tissue common after surgery.

Long-term prognosis
A large percentage of athletes may be unable to continue sports following a shoulder dislocation without subsequent injuries or the need for surgical treatment. Furthermore, athletes who undergo surgery following shoulder dislocation are often unable to perform at their former level. The alternative method of prolotherapy may offer relief and more effective healing.

SHOULDER SUBLUXATION

The shoulder complex enables extreme mobility due to its anatomical structure but provides little stability. Glenohumeral subluxation is a partial dislocation of the ball-and-socket joint of the shoulder. Instability in the shoulder joint complex, particularly following dislocation, can result in subluxation.

Cause of injury
A direct blow to the shoulder. A fall onto an outstretched arm. Strenuously forcing the arm into an awkward position.

Signs and symptoms
Sensation of the shoulder going in and out of the joint. Looseness of the shoulder joint. Pain, weakness or numbness in the shoulder or arm.

Complications if left unattended
Untreated subluxation can cause wear and ultimately damage to the internal structures of the shoulder, sometimes requiring surgery. Loss of mobility, ongoing pain and osteoarthritic complications may result from untreated subluxation.

Immediate treatment
RICER regimen to reduce inflammation and treat pain. Anti-inflammatory medicines and analgesics for pain.

Rehabilitation and prevention
Following immobilization and healing, strengthening exercises should be undertaken. Recovery depends on factors including the athlete's age, health, history of previous injury and severity of subluxation. If the shoulder subluxates frequently during activity, significant physical rehabilitation will be needed and possibly surgery.

Long-term prognosis
Normal sports activity may be resumed once a full range of motion without subluxation has been achieved. Prognosis is dependent on the severity of the subluxation and the athlete's particular history. Subluxation is often due to previous shoulder injury and returning to athletics before full recovery can lead to further and worsening instability.

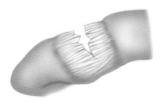

ACROMIOCLAVICULAR SEPARATION

Acromioclavicular separation is a rupture of the ligaments that connect the clavicle to the tip of the scapula known as the acromion process. Acromioclavicular (AC) joint injuries generally occur in the course of upper-extremity strength training, various throwing sports and collision sports (particularly football and hockey). The injury is common among athletes in their 30s and 40s.

Cause of injury
Fall onto the point of the shoulder. Fall onto an outstretched hand. Direct blow to the shoulder.

Signs and symptoms
Pain, tenderness and swelling at the AC joint. Deformity of the injured joint. Pain or discomfort during cross-body adduction (turning the injured arm inward toward the opposite shoulder).

Complications if left unattended
Degenerative joint abnormalities, chronic pain and stiffness and limitations in mobility requiring surgery are possible should the condition not be given prompt medical attention and allowed proper healing time.

Immediate treatment
Immobilization of the injured arm with a sling. Ice packs, rest and the use of anti-inflammatory medication and analgesics for pain.

Rehabilitation and prevention
AC separations of a less severe nature are successfully treated without surgery, though a thorough healing period of 6–8 weeks is generally required. Following this, range-of-motion exercises should be used to avoid stiffness. Exercises directed at maintaining strength and stability of the shoulder and upper back muscles may help prevent the injury, and use of padding around the AC joint, particularly during contact sports, may help avoid re-injury.

Long-term prognosis
Given adequate healing time and rehabilitation, most AC separations are resolved without surgery. Should surgery be required, risks of infection and continued pain exist, and recovery time for the athlete is lengthened.

STERNOCLAVICULAR SEPARATION

Sternoclavicular separation occurs when a ligament connecting the clavicle to the sternum is torn. Rotation at the joint is affected by this injury, which may occur during contact sports when the shoulder forcefully strikes the ground or is landed on by another player. The separation may occur anteriorly or posteriorly (in front of or behind the sternum).

Cause of injury

Direct blow to the sternum. Fall onto the shoulder or outstretched hands. Shoulder striking the ground, or another athlete landing on top of the shoulder.

Signs and symptoms

Pain, swelling and tenderness over the SC joint. Abnormal movement between the sternum and clavicle. Possible displacement of the clavicle in front of or behind the sternum.

Complications if left unattended

Untreated sternoclavicular separation can lead to loss of motion and ongoing pain, stiffness and weakness around the shoulder. In cases where the clavicle is forced behind the breastbone the risk exists for damage to important underlying blood vessels requiring surgical intervention.

Immediate treatment

Reduction of the joint where needed and immobilization with a sling. RICER to reduce swelling, trauma and pain.

Rehabilitation and prevention

As the injury is generally caused in sports accidents, prevention is usually not possible. In the case of anterior injury to the SC joint (the most common), the condition is generally resolved without permanent complications given adequate healing time. In more severe cases, surgery may be required. Range of motion exercises should help restore movement and rotational ability.

Long-term prognosis

With adequate time for healing, the injured athlete typically makes a full recovery. If the injury is serious (particularly in the case of posterior dislocation) instability of the joint may persist, in some cases requiring surgery.

BICEPS BRACHII TENDON RUPTURE

Repetitive strain, particularly due to over-lifting, can lead to irritation and microscopic tears in the biceps brachii tendon, which connects the biceps brachii muscle to the scapula at the proximal end and the radius and fascia of the forearm at the distal end. A biceps brachii tendon rupture results from sudden trauma to the biceps brachii tendon. Injury at the proximal end of the tendon of the long head of biceps is most common. Biceps brachii tendon ruptures can occur from weight lifting or throwing sports but are generally uncommon, particularly in young athletes. In older individuals it is often the result of degenerative change or previous injury to the tendon.

Cause of injury
Weakness due to tears in the rotator cuff. Throwing activities. Weightlifting.

Signs and symptoms
Bulge in the upper arm. Inability to turn the palm upward. Sudden, sharp pain at the shoulder.

Complications if left unattended
Generally, little functional loss accompanies rupture of a proximal biceps brachii tendon, as two tendinous attachments occur at the shoulder, one compensating the other in most cases. For this reason, surgery is rarely required and complications are rare, though without proper healing, re-tearing and degeneration of the tendon are more likely.

Immediate treatment
Anti-inflammatory and analgesic medications to reduce pain. RICER regimen immediately following injury. Later heat to promote blood flow and healing.

Rehabilitation and prevention
Following rest and recovery of the tendon, flexibility and strengthening exercises should be undertaken to restore full mobility in the shoulder. Avoidance of sudden lifting beyond normal capacity and violent loading to the biceps brachii tendon as during throwing sports may help prevent the injury.

Long-term prognosis
Most biceps brachii tendon ruptures resolve without medical intervention if given proper time for healing. In younger athletes with demanding training schedules, surgery may be contemplated to repair the rupture. Tears and ruptures to the distal end of the biceps brachii tendon at the elbow are more rare but can be more severe, requiring surgery. In both cases the prospects for full recovery are excellent.

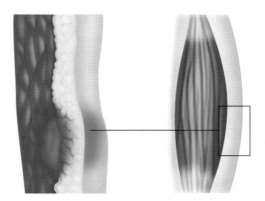

BICEPS BRACHII BRUISE

Bruising to the biceps brachii can occur following tearing and/or rupture of the tendon or trauma to the muscle. Overstrain from weight training can cause tears and bruising which may also result from throwing sports or following direct trauma to the shoulder during a fall or collision with another athlete.

Cause of injury
Direct blow to the biceps brachii region of the upper arm. Biceps brachii tendon rupture. Repetitive strain to the biceps brachii muscle or tendon.

Signs and symptoms
Discolouration of the biceps brachii area. Aching or tenderness in the muscle. Stiffness and limitation of movement in the affected arm and shoulder.

Complications if left unattended
Bruising of the biceps brachii generally resolves without treatment. Sports involving heavy use of the biceps brachii muscle including weight training and throwing sports and contact activities with high risk to the biceps brachii should be avoided to give adequate time for healing.

Immediate treatment
RICER regimen and analgesics to reduce inflammation and pain. Immobilization with a sling to prevent excess movement.

Rehabilitation and prevention
Rest and avoidance of activities involving stress to the biceps brachii muscle and tendons during the healing phase are generally sufficient. Range of motion exercises and graded strength training should be undertaken to restore full power and resilience to the muscle. Stretching exercises performed before athletic activity may help prevent injury and associated bruising.

Long-term prognosis
Bruising to biceps brachii is generally a minor condition that is self-correcting without resort to surgery, given adequate time for healing. No long-term deficit in strength or mobility is expected.

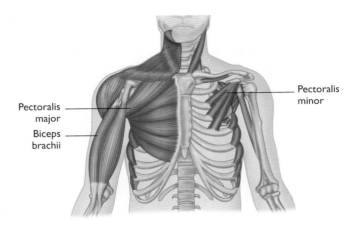

Pectoralis major

Biceps brachii

Pectoralis minor

MUSCLE STRAIN (BICEPS BRACHII, PECTORAL MUSCLES)

Muscle strains are among the most common sports injuries and often result from the sudden extension of a joint beyond its normal range. This causes damage to muscle and other soft tissue. The chest muscles (pectoralis major and minor) join the biceps brachii muscle at the shoulder. Weight training, sudden, violent torsion of the shoulder during throwing sports or sudden force applied to the nexus of the pectorals and biceps brachii (as when warding off a check in hockey with the arm extended) can produce such injuries.

Cause of injury
Sudden movement leading to a muscle tear. Large physical demand placed on the muscle. Warding off a check in hockey or tackle in football.

Signs and symptoms
Tenderness and pain over the affected muscle. Stiffness. Pain during muscle use.

Complications if left unattended
Muscle strains are usually self-limiting and repair themselves given proper time off from exertion for healing. Insufficient recovery time can lead to further tearing, increasing the risk of re-injury and cause degenerative changes in the muscles over time.

Immediate treatment
RICER regimen and analgesics to reduce inflammation and pain. Then heat to promote blood flow and healing.

Rehabilitation and prevention
Stretching exercises following healing can help restore full mobility to the affected area while strengthening exercises can help prevent re-injury. Stretching and warm-up, as well as attention to proper athletic technique (particularly in weight training) may help prevent this type of injury.

Long-term prognosis
Muscle strains involving the pectoral muscles and / or biceps brachii are common and – given adequate time for proper healing – generally not a serious threat to the athlete, although severe or repeated muscle strains can cause chronic pain and lead to impairment of muscle function.

047: MUSCLE STRAIN (BICEPS BRACHII, CHEST)

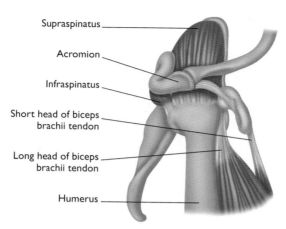

Supraspinatus

Acromion

Infraspinatus

Short head of biceps
brachii tendon

Long head of biceps
brachii tendon

Humerus

SUBACROMIAL IMPINGEMENT

Subacromial impingement problems in the athlete are associated with repetitive overhead activity and throwing events. Compression of the narrow subacromial space on the top of the shoulder between the head of the humerus and the acromion of the scapula results in local pain and loss of coordination in the rotator cuff muscles of the shoulder. Tissue trauma associated with it includes damage to the glenoid labrum, the tendon of the long head of biceps brachii and the subacromial bursa. Dysfunction and damage in the muscles of the rotator cuff can cause the humeral head to displace upward during elevation of the arm, leading to irritation of structures in the subacromial space such as the supraspinatus tendon and subacromial bursa.

Cause of injury
Repeated overhead movements as in tennis, swimming, golf and weightlifting. Irritation of the rotator cuff due to throwing sports including baseball. Underlying predisposition, including rheumatoid arthritis.

Signs and symptoms
Shoulder pain and difficulty raising the arm in the air. Pain during sleep when the injured arm is rolled on. Pain during rotational movements such as reaching into a back pocket.

Complications if left unattended
Increasing stiffness of the joint and further loss of motion may result should impingement be ignored. Rotator cuff tendons may be torn should athletic activity be undertaken prior to full recovery. Tendinitis and bursitis frequently develop with impingement as a pre-condition.

Immediate treatment
Rest, ice packs and anti-inflammatory medication. Corticosteroid injections may be used under the acromion to reduce inflammation.

Rehabilitation and prevention
Following a period of healing, physical therapy will often be used to restore strength and range of motion in the affected rotator cuff. Avoiding or limiting repetitive motions that cause rotator cuff irritation may help prevent the injury. Strengthening exercises and light-weight training to strengthen the muscles of the rotator cuff are also useful preventive measures.

Long-term prognosis
Typically, the condition shows marked improvement within 6–12 weeks. In cases where recovery has not been achieved in 6–12 months, surgery may be recommended to release the ligaments. Surgery is usually followed by physical therapy, and some modification of athletic activity may be necessary to reduce the chances of relapse.

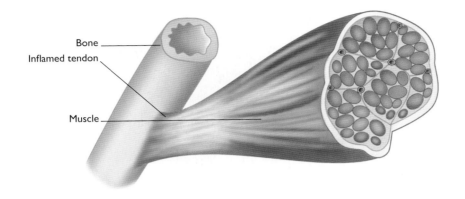

Bone
Inflamed tendon
Muscle

ROTATOR CUFF TENDINITIS

Rotator cuff tendinitis results from the irritation and inflammation of the tendons of the rotator cuff muscles in the area underlying the acromion. The condition is sometimes known as pitcher's shoulder though it is a common injury in all sports requiring overhead arm movements, including tennis, volleyball, swimming and weightlifting.

Cause of injury
Inflammation of the rotator cuff tendons from tennis, baseball, swimming etc. Irritation of the subacromial bursa of the rotator cuff causing inflammation and swelling in the subacromial space. Pre-existing disposition including anatomical irregularity.

Signs and symptoms
Weakness or pain with overhead activities, such as brushing hair, reaching up etc. Popping or cracking sensation in the shoulder. Pain in the injured shoulder, particularly when lying on it.

Complications if left unattended
Rotator cuff tendinitis can worsen without attention as the tendons and bursa become increasingly inflamed. Motion becomes more limited and tendon tears can cause further and in some cases chronic pain. Prolonged irritation may result in the production of bone spurs which contribute to further irritation.

Immediate treatment
Application of ice and use of anti-inflammatory medication. Discontinue all athletic and other activity causing rotator cuff pain. Then heat to promote blood flow and healing.

Rehabilitation and prevention
Following rest and healing of the injured shoulder, physical therapy should be undertaken to strengthen the muscles of the rotator cuff. Occasionally steroid injections are required to reduce pain and inflammation. Moderation of rotator cuff use, adequate recovery time between athletic activities and strength training can all help avoid the injury.

Long-term prognosis
Given proper rest as well as physical therapy and (where needed) steroidal injections, most athletes enjoy a full recovery from this injury. Should a serious tear of the rotator cuff tissue occur, surgery may be required although recovery to pre-injury levels of activity is usually expected.

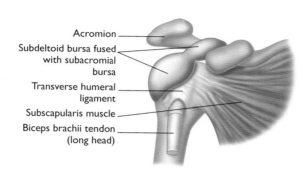

Acromion
Subdeltoid bursa fused with subacromial bursa
Transverse humeral ligament
Subscapularis muscle
Biceps brachii tendon (long head)

SHOULDER BURSITIS

Shoulder bursitis is not generally an isolated condition but is usually associated with a rotator cuff tear or impingement syndrome. The subacromial bursa is the largest and most commonly injured bursa in the shoulder region.

Bursitis may be caused by a combination of factors including rotator cuff dysfunction, instability in the joints of the pectoral girdle, osteoarthritis, postural misalignments, bone spurs and anything that decreases space in the limited subacromial space.

Cause of injury
Overuse from throwing activities, tennis, swimming or baseball. Falling onto an outstretched arm. Local infection.

Signs and symptoms
Pain in the shoulder, particularly when raising the arm. Pain on lying on or compressing the injured shoulder. Loss of strength and limited motion of the shoulder.

Complications if left unattended
Failure to attend to shoulder bursitis generally results in a worsening of the condition, a further thickening of tendons and bursa(e) leading to increased inflammation and pain. The athlete runs the risk of developing a chronic condition, as well as a danger that the fluid in the bursa(e) becomes infected, a potentially serious situation sometimes necessitating surgery.

Immediate treatment
Discontinue all activity causing inflammation of the shoulder. RICER regimen and analgesics to reduce inflammation and pain. Then heat to promote blood flow and healing.

Rehabilitation and prevention
The athlete should avoid pressure to the injured shoulder and inflamed bursa(e) during recovery as well as any activities likely to irritate the condition. Begin exercising the shoulder when instructed by a medical professional in order to restore strength and shoulder mobility. Warming-up and cooling-down exercises, with an emphasis on stretching, strength training and maintaining looseness in the shoulder can help prevent bursitis from developing.

Long-term prognosis
Shoulder bursitis tends to ease with proper healing and minor rehabilitation, and a full recovery to athletic activity can usually be expected, particularly if no infection of the bursa is present. In some cases, aspiration of bursal fluid by needle is recommended to reduce inflammation and ensure no infection is present.

BICIPITAL TENDINITIS

Bicipital tendinitis results from irritation and inflammation to the biceps brachii tendon, which lies on the front of the shoulder and allows elbow flexion and supination of the forearm. Overuse can lead to inflammation and is a common affliction in golfers, weightlifters, rowers and those engaged in throwing sports.

Irritation of the tendon of the long head of biceps occurs as it moves up and down in the intertubercular (bicipital) groove of the humerus. Inflammation can be to the tendon itself or to the tendon sheath or paratenons. The musculo-tendinous junction of biceps brachii is highly susceptible to injuries brought on by overuse, particularly following repetitive lifting activities.

Cause of injury
Poor technique, particularly in weightlifting. Sudden increase in duration or intensity of training. Shoulder impingement syndrome.

Signs and symptoms
Pain over the bicipital groove when the tendon is passively stretched and during resisted supination and elbow flexion. Pain and tenderness along the tendon length. Stiffness following exercise.

Complications if left unattended
Bicipital tendinitis, left without care and treatment, generally worsens as the biceps brachii tendon becomes increasingly irritated and inflamed. Movement and the ability to perform athletically without pain will be further hampered. Exercising without adequate healing and rehabilitation can lead to tearing of the tendon and tendon degeneration over time.

Immediate treatment
RICER regimen to relieve painful inflammation. Anti-inflammatory and analgesic medication. Then heat to promote blood flow and healing.

Rehabilitation and prevention
The condition is self-limiting given rest and minimal medical attention. Following full recovery, exercises directed at improving flexibility, proprioception and strength may be undertaken. Thorough warm-up and stretching exercises and a steady athletic regimen that avoids sudden, unprepared increases in activity can help avoid this injury, as can attention to proper sports technique.

Long-term prognosis
A full return to athletic activity may generally be expected given adequate time for tendon recovery and reduction of inflammation. However, the injury frequently recurs. Surgery is generally not required. Corticosteroid injections are sometimes used to reduce pain, though they must be applied cautiously as they increase the risk of tendon rupture.

PECTORAL MUSCLE INSERTION INFLAMMATION

The pectoralis major or pectoral muscle is used in many sports when the arms act to push away a weight (as during weightlifting) or another athlete (during various contact sports). Repetitive activity, particularly bench-pressing, can cause irritation to the muscle and/or tendon leading to discomfort and loss of mobility.

Cause of injury
Excessive load on the pectoralis major muscle, especially when bench-pressing. Excessive force against the muscle from pushing activities in contact sports. A fall onto one or both outstretched arms.

Signs and symptoms
Pain and weakness in the shoulder. Difficulty raising the arm. Pain or stiffness during lifting.

Complications if left unattended
Irritation of the pectoral muscle insertion will become further aggravated if it is neglected. Tears in the muscle or tendon can develop, leading to increased pain and weakness and the danger of long-term degeneration of muscle and tendon. Should tearing at the insertion point become serious, surgery may be required to repair it.

Immediate treatment
Immediate cessation to athletic activity causing irritation. RICER regimen to reduce inflammation and treat pain. Then heat to promote blood flow and healing.

Rehabilitation and prevention
Thorough healing time must be allowed for the pectoral muscle and associated tendons. Strength training of the pectorals through weights and graded calisthenics will generally help restore the athlete to prior condition, provided no serious tearing of the muscle has resulted. Attention to proper weight training technique and a gradual rather than sudden increase in stress on the pectoral muscles can help prevent this injury.

Long-term prognosis
Given proper care and healing time, combined with gradual strength training of the pectoral and shoulder muscle complex, the athlete may generally expect a full return to normal activity.

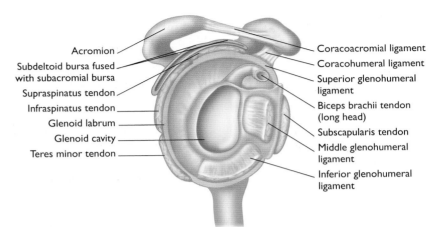

Acromion
Subdeltoid bursa fused with subacromial bursa
Supraspinatus tendon
Infraspinatus tendon
Glenoid labrum
Glenoid cavity
Teres minor tendon

Coracoacromial ligament
Coracohumeral ligament
Superior glenohumeral ligament
Biceps brachii tendon (long head)
Subscapularis tendon
Middle glenohumeral ligament
Inferior glenohumeral ligament

FROZEN SHOULDER (ADHESIVE CAPSULITIS)

Frozen shoulder or adhesive capsulitis causes severe restriction of shoulder movement due to pain. The condition results from abnormal bands of tissue that form on the joint capsule, thereby restricting motion and producing pain on movement. Synovial fluid which usually serves to lubricate the joint space allowing smooth motion is often lacking in this condition. Idiopathic adhesive capsulitis is more common in females and diabetics. Onset in the athlete may follow trauma to the shoulder.

Cause of injury
Scar tissue formation following shoulder injury. Formation of adhesions following shoulder surgery. Repeated tearing of soft tissue surrounding the glenohumeral joint.

Signs and symptoms
Dull, aching pain in the shoulder region, often worse at night. Restricted movement of the shoulder. Pain when moving the affected arm.

Complications if left unattended
Frozen shoulder has a tendency to worsen over time without adequate treatment and proper recovery period. Attempted athletic activity involving the affected shoulder will likely lead to further adhesions of the joint, with further pain and restrictions of movement. Production of scar tissue may eventually require surgical removal.

Immediate treatment
Application of moist heat to the shoulder to loosen the affected joint. Muscle relaxants to relax shoulder muscles and arm.

Rehabilitation and prevention
Moist heat should be accompanied by stretching exercises to gradually restore mobility. Heat therapy should be combined with doctor-supervised physical therapy. Moving the shoulder through the full range of motion several times daily, as well as strength training exercises, may help avoid frozen shoulder. Injuries to the shoulder should be given prompt medical attention to avoid formation of scar tissue where possible.

Long-term prognosis
The length of recovery time following frozen shoulder varies depending on the underlying cause as well as the age and health of the athlete and the history of shoulder injury. If the condition fails to improve after 4–6 months surgery may be required. Some lasting discomfort and impairment of movement is common with this injury.

REHABILITATION EXERCISES

Standing dumbbell press

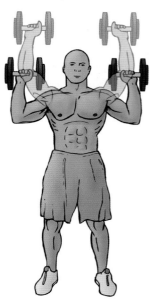

Grip dumbbells with your palms facing forward and the dumbbells level with your ears. Press them upwards toward the ceiling and then bring the dumbbells down slowly without letting them fall past your ears and repeat.

Alternate front raise

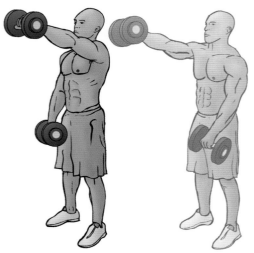

Grip a dumbbell in each hand letting them rest on the tops of your thighs. Raise one dumbbell while keeping your palm facing the floor. Lower the dumbbell to the start position and repeat with the other arm.

Lateral raise

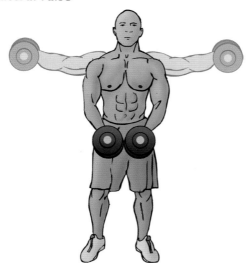

Grip a dumbbell in each hand with your palms facing each other. Simultaneously raise your arms out to the side so that your palms face the ground. Lower the dumbbells to the start position and repeat.

Alternate dumbbell curl

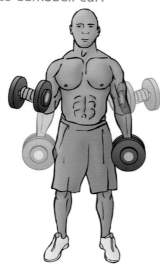

Grip a dumbbell in each hand and let them fall naturally at your sides. Lift one at a time by bending your elbow and raising the dumbbell toward your chest. Slowly lower the dumbbell to the start position and repeat with the other arm.

Press-ups

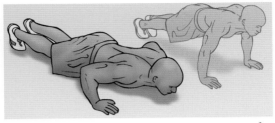

Lie face down with your palms on the floor positioned slightly to the side of your shoulders. Raise your body up by pressing against the floor until your elbows are straight. Slowly lower your body until your chest grazes the floor and repeat.

Reach back shoulder stretch

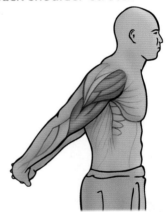

Stand upright and clasp your hands together behind your back. Slowly lift your hands upward.

Wall-assisted chest stretch

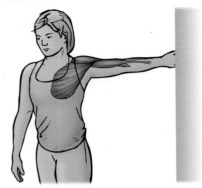

Stand with your arm extended to the rear and parallel to the ground. Hold on to an immovable object and then turn your shoulders and body away from your outstretched arm.

Sports Injuries of the Back and Spine

ANATOMY AND PHYSIOLOGY

The spine (vertebral column) is made up of bones known as vertebrae, separated by fibrocartilage intervertebral discs. The spine consists of 33 vertebrae in total: 7 cervical, 12 thoracic, 5 lumbar (the largest weightbearing vertebrae), 5 (fused) sacral and 3–4 (fused) in the coccyx (tailbone). There is only slight movement between any two successive vertebrae, but there is considerable movement throughout the spinal column as a whole. The intervertebral discs are composed of a thick ring of fibrous cartilage known as the annulus fibrosis which surrounds a jelly-like material known as the nucleus pulposus. Intervertebral discs provide flexibility, cushioning and protection to the spine. The spinal canal runs through the center of the vertebrae posterior to the discs and contains the spinal cord running from the brain stem to the level of the first or second lumbar vertebrae.

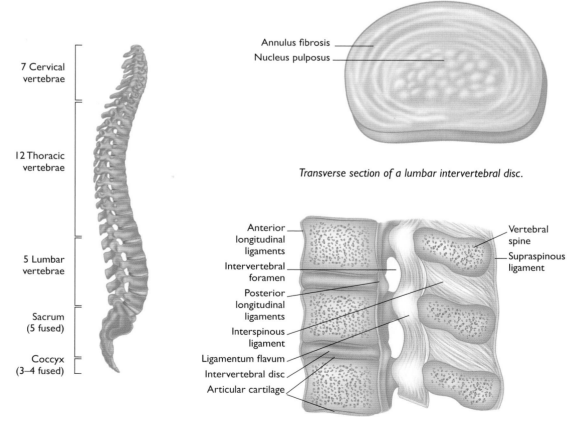

Transverse section of a lumbar intervertebral disc.

The vertebral column, lateral view.

Sagittal section of vertebra.

Ligaments are resilient bands made up of fibrous tissue. They provide strong, flexible linkages between bones. A number of ligaments support the spine. The anterior and posterior longitudinal ligaments connect the vertebral bodies in the cervical, thoracic and lumbar regions. The supraspinous ligament attaches to the spinous processes of the vertebrae. It is enlarged in the cervical region where it is known as the ligamentum nuchae. The ligamenta flava attach to, and extend between, the ventral portions of the laminae of two adjacent vertebrae, from C2/C3 to L5/S1. The ligaments, muscles and tendons work together to manage external forces to the spine during movement, particularly bending and lifting.

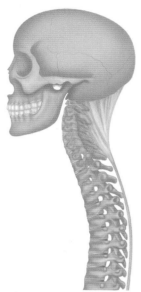

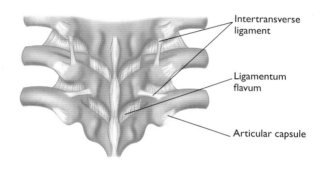

Intertransverse ligament

Ligamentum flavum

Articular capsule

Ligamentum nuchae.

A typical vertebral arch joint, posterior view.

The muscles around the spine are primarily responsible for stabilizing the spinal column and keeping the back in an upright position. The muscles of the back and sides allow the upper body and spine to move in flexion, lateral flexion, extension, hyperextension and rotation.

Latissimus dorsi, the broadest muscle of the back, is one of the chief climbing muscles, since it pulls the shoulders downwards and backwards, and pulls the trunk up to the fixed arms. It is therefore heavily used in sports such as climbing, gymnastics (in particular rings and parallel bars), swimming and rowing. The rhomboid muscles are situated between the scapula and vertebral column, and are so named because of their shape (rhombus). Quadratus lumborum runs across the waist from the iliac crest and iliolumbar ligament up to the lowest rib and the transverse processes of L1 to L4. Its action is to side-bend the trunk and also to resist the trunk being pulled sideways in the opposite direction.

The intercostal muscles are thin, layered sheets of muscle running between adjacent ribs. The external intercostal muscles of the lower ribs may blend with the fibres of external oblique muscles of the abdomen, which overlap them, thus effectively forming one continuous sheet of muscle. Internal intercostal fibres lie deep to, and run obliquely across, the external intercostals.

The erector spinae muscles of the back , also called sacrospinalis, comprise three sets of muscles organised in parallel columns. From lateral to medial, they are: iliocostalis, longissimus and spinalis. Longissimus is the intermediate part of the erector spinae. It may be subdivided into thoracis, cervicis and capitis portions. The spinalis is the most medial part of the erector spinae. It may be subdivided into thoracis, cervicis and capitis portions.

The transversospinalis muscles are a composite of three small muscle groups situated deep to the erector spinae. Unlike the erector spinae, each group lies successively deeper rather than side by side. The muscle groups are, from superficial to deep: semispinalis, multifidus and rotatores. Their fibres generally extend upward and medially from transverse processes to higher spinous processes. Multifidus is the part of the transversospinalis group that lies in the furrow between the spines of the vertebrae and their transverse processes. It lies deep to semispinalis and the erector spinae. Rotatores are the deepest layer of the transversospinalis group.

Interspinales are short and insignificant muscles positioned either side of the interspinous ligament. Like the interspinales, the intertransversarii are also short and insignificant muscles. The cervical and thoracic regions encompass intertransversarii anteriores and intertransversarii posteriores, and the lumbar region encompasses intertransversarii laterales and intertransversarii mediales.

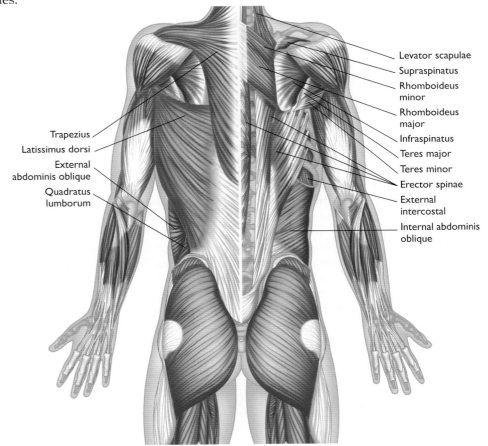

Levator scapulae
Supraspinatus
Rhomboideus minor
Rhomboideus major
Infraspinatus
Teres major
Teres minor
Erector spinae
External intercostal
Internal abdominis oblique

Trapezius
Latissimus dorsi
External abdominis oblique
Quadratus lumborum

Muscles of the back.

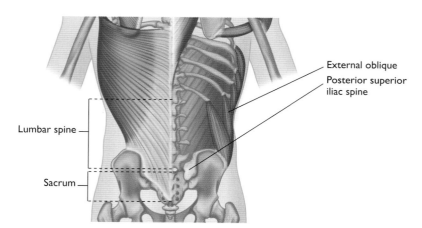

External oblique

Posterior superior iliac spine

Lumbar spine

Sacrum

MUSCLE STRAIN OF THE BACK

Back strain frequently involves the lower back (lumbar spine and sacrum). Back strain occurs from a stretching injury to the muscles or tendons of the back. It is a common sports injury that can result from lifting, sudden movement, or a fall, collision with another athlete, or any activity in which the muscles of the back are engaged. Back strain often affects the lower back or lumbar region and the pain associated with this injury ranges from moderate to severe.

Cause of injury
Sudden strain on the back muscles from lifting. Abrupt movement involving muscles of the back. Repetitive stress to the back muscles. Poor technique or postural weakness.

Signs and symptoms
Pain, stiffness and loss of movement in the back.

Complications if left unattended
Muscle strains in the back usually resolve with proper rest. Ignoring muscle strain, however, can lead to chronic back pain, stiffness and discomfort, with degeneration of the muscles and tendons. Muscle spasms accompanying inflammation can cause further pain, in some cases severe.

Immediate treatment
Rest on a firm surface, lying on the back with knees raised rather than on the stomach. Ice pack, analgesic and anti-inflammatory medication.

Rehabilitation and prevention
After use of ice to reduce inflammation, heat therapy in modest amounts may help ease discomfort. Recovery times for muscle strain in the back vary widely depending on the severity of the strain, location and overall health of the athlete. When the muscles have begun to heal, it is important that they receive moderate use to avoid wasting and atrophy. Later, exercises to strengthen the back and restore mobility can help avoid recurrence of this injury.

Long-term prognosis
Muscle strains in the back, though sometimes quite painful, usually heal thoroughly with no residual loss of movement or pain, though some risk of re-injury exists, particularly if the strain was severe. Surgery is not required in cases of muscle strain, provided no severe tearing of tissue or tendon is involved.

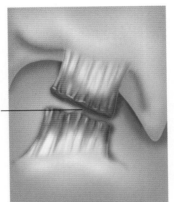

Ruptured ligament

LIGAMENT SPRAIN OF THE BACK

Sudden, irregular motion, repetitive stress or excessive load on the ligaments associated with the spine can cause a sprain or tearing of the ligaments. The resulting injury, which affects athletes in a broad variety of sports, produces pain and varying degrees of immobility.

Cause of injury

Lifting beyond normal capacity. Sudden torsion of the spine, including a fall during skiing or other sport. Unprepared movement involving the back.

Signs and symptoms

Pain and stiffness. Difficulty bending over and pain when straightening the back. Tenderness and inflammation.

Complications if left unattended

A sprain to the ligaments will generally force the athlete to rest the injury and allow healing time due to pain and stiffness precluding normal activity. Should activity be continued before adequate healing, further tearing of the ligaments and lasting ligament injury may result. A mild ligament sprain can become acutely painful and incapacitating if ignored.

Immediate treatment

RICER regimen immediately following injury. Non-steroidal anti-inflammatory drugs (NSAIDs).

Rehabilitation and prevention

In the case of mild to moderate ligament sprain, a few days' rest should allow a return to most non-athletic daily activity. This should be undertaken to re-establish flexibility in the spine and avoid atrophy. Strengthening exercises for the back should not be undertaken until full recovery. Warm-ups and stretching prior to sports, good posture and attention to proper technique can help avoid this injury.

Long-term prognosis

Less than 5% of back injuries require surgery, and surgery is rarely warranted for ligament sprain, although 6–8 weeks of recovery are often required, sometimes longer, should the sprain be serious. Failure to allow complete healing will increase the risk of re-injury.

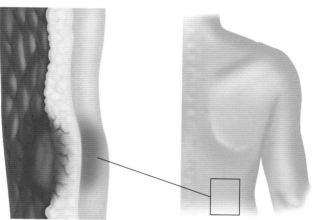

THORACIC CONTUSION

A contusion is a closed wound to the body's soft tissue, resulting from a blow to muscle, tendon or ligament. Contusion injuries cause bruising and often discolouration due to blood pooling around the site of trauma. Contusions of the back are possible in a variety of contact sports such as football and hockey due to violent force applied to the soft tissues or as the result of a fall onto the back.

Contusions involve trauma to the subcutaneous tissue. Because the musculature is well vascularized and the regional blood flow is usually high at the moment of impact, bleeding occurs from torn blood vessels into the skin and subcutaneous tissues, forming a bruise or ecchymosis (discolouration of an area of the skin). Capillaries are damaged due to blunt force, resulting in blood seeping into the surrounding tissue. While most contusions acquired in the course of sports activity are minor, some are symptomatic of serious injuries including fractures or internal bleeding.

Cause of injury
Overloading or over-stretching muscles through a blow to the back from another athlete during contact sports. Blow from sports equipment, especially hockey and lacrosse. Hard fall onto the back.

Signs and symptoms
Pain at injury site. Tenderness to the touch. Blue, purple, orange or yellow discolouration of the skin. Painful spasms and knot-like contractions (which act as a protective mechanism).

Complications if left unattended
Contusions may indicate more serious underlying conditions including fracture, haematoma (blood in the muscle) or other internal bleeding, all of which should receive prompt medical attention. Minor contusions generally clear up in a matter of days without complication. More severe cases, however, may require 3–4 weeks to heal.

Immediate treatment
Discontinue activity and apply ice to reduce swelling. Anti-inflammatory medication and analgesics for pain, if needed. Activity modification.

Rehabilitation and prevention
Avoiding pressure or further trauma to the contusion site and application of ice are usually sufficient to speed recovery. As contusions result from blunt force accidents, they are generally not preventable, though proper conditioning and diet (including an abundance of vitamin C) may lessen the severity of contusion. Follow-up management may include application of superficial heat, ultrasound, massage and appropriate stretching and resistance exercise.

Long-term prognosis
While contusions in the back can produce significant acute pain, they are faster to heal than muscle strains or ligament sprains. Severity of bruising depends on many factors, including muscle tension or relaxation at the time of injury. Pain will generally subside in hours or days and skin discolouration will abate as well. The athlete should enjoy a full return to activity, in more severe cases after about 4 weeks, without lasting deficit.

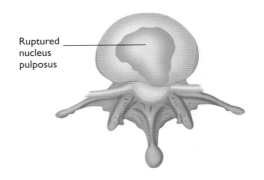

Ruptured nucleus pulposus

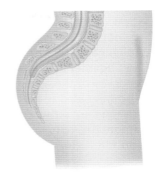

DISC PROLAPSE

Discs are segments of connective tissue that separate the vertebrae of the spine, providing absorption from shock and allowing for the smooth flexing of the neck and back without the vertebral bones rubbing against each other.

A slipped disc (also known as a herniated, ruptured or prolapsed disc) results when the shock-absorbing pads or intervertebral discs split or rupture. The discs contain a jelly-like substance which seeps out into the surrounding tissue, causing local inflammation and pressure on the spinal nerves (and occasionally the spinal cord) where they exit the spinal canal. Slipped discs most frequently occur in the lower back although any disc of the spine is vulnerable to rupture.

Cause of injury
Improper weightlifting technique. Excessive strain. Forceful trauma to the vertebral disc.

Signs and symptoms
Pain in the back or neck. Numbness, tingling or pain in the buttocks, back, upper or lower limb. Changes in bowel or bladder function (this is rare but should be treated as a medical emergency).

Complications if left unattended
Slipped or herniated discs require medical attention and evaluation. Symptoms of slipped disc may indicate other underlying ailments including fracture, tumours, infection or nerve damage, with serious – in certain cases, life-threatening – implications.

Immediate treatment
Bed rest, application of alternating ice and heat. Use of anti-inflammatory and analgesic medication.

Rehabilitation and prevention
Rest and limited activity for several days is usually indicated, though normal, non-athletic daily activity should be resumed soon thereafter to prevent atrophy and restore mobility in the spine. Physical therapy may be combined with massage and gradually increasing exercise of the back after the pain has subsided. Strengthening and flexibility exercises, proper warm-up, avoidance of excessive or sudden weight lifting and attention to good sports technique may help avoid the injury.

Long-term prognosis
Most disc injuries are resolved without surgery, given proper recovery time. Though full restoration of strength and mobility may generally be expected, discs are vulnerable to re-injury, particularly for weightlifters and athletes placing significant demands on the back muscles, tendons and ligaments and on the spine itself.

DISC BULGE

A bulging disc is one that has extended outward beyond its normal boundary due to various forms of degeneration. Should the disc impinge on the ligaments connecting the vertebrae or on nerves of the spine, pain results. A bulging disc may also result when the nucleus pulposus pushes outward. Disc bulges may be asymptomatic, only appearing on a magnetic resonance imaging (MRI) scan.

Cause of injury
Age-related wear and degeneration. Stretching of ligaments connecting vertebrae. Successive strains from improper weight training.

Signs and symptoms
Back pain radiating to the legs (lumbar discs). Back pain radiating to the shoulders (cervical discs). Numbness, tingling or pain in the buttocks, back, upper or lower limb.

Complications if left unattended
A bulging disc may not cause symptoms and may not be diagnosed without a medical scan. As a disc bulges more over time, however, it may begin to impinge on nerves and cause pain. Sudden stress to the discs, as during abrupt movements or weightlifting, can cause rupture or herniation of the disc, a more painful condition requiring rest and rehabilitation.

Immediate treatment
Cessation of activity stressing the spinal discs. Rest and alternating ice and heat to reduce inflammation and pain.

Rehabilitation and prevention
Bulging discs often occur as a natural consequence of the aging process, though in some cases they are a precursor to disc herniation or rupture. Bulging discs are an example of contained injury while herniated discs are considered uncontained. Minimizing undue stress on the back may help avoid this injury.

Long-term prognosis
More severely bulging discs may in time rupture, causing the inner material to extrude into the spinal canal. In less severe cases, rest and ice are generally sufficient to restore pain-free mobility to the athlete.

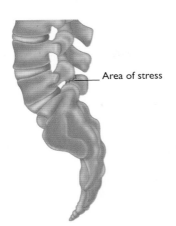

Area of stress

STRESS FRACTURE OF THE VERTEBRA

The upper and lower joints of the lumbar spine are joined by the pars interarticularis, the weakest bony portion of the vertebral neural arch, and the region between the superior and inferior articular facets. Overuse injuries can result in cracks or fractures in the pars interarticularis, sometimes to the point where the vertebrae shift out of place; this condition is known as spondylolisthesis. The lowest lumbar vertebra (L5), where the spine meets the pelvis, is the most common site for vertebral fractures.

Stress fractures of the vertebrae (spondylolysis) are a common athletic injury caused by overuse or hyperextension of the spine. Gymnastics, weightlifting and football are among the sports prone to this injury, and it is a particularly common occurrence in adolescent athletes during sudden growth spurts.

Cause of injury
Genetic predisposition. Mechanical stress caused by overuse, flexion, twisting or hyperextension of the lumbar spine. Growth spurts, especially in adolescents.

Signs and symptoms
Pain spreading across the lower back. Spasms causing stiffening in the back. Tightening of hamstring muscles, causing changes in posture.

Complications if left unattended
If slippage due to vertebral fracture is ignored, it will worsen and can become incapacitating. Bone that has developed cracks requires sufficient time to rebuild, a process known as remodeling. Surgery may ultimately be required should fractures further develop and become severe.

Immediate treatment
Rest and avoidance of overuse or stress to the lumbar vertebrae. Ice pack, analgesic and anti-inflammatory drugs to reduce inflammation and pain. Then heat to promote blood flow and healing.

Rehabilitation and prevention
Following a thorough healing period (which may last 6 weeks or longer depending on the severity of injury), flexibility and strength training exercises should be undertaken, avoiding overuse. Exercising on hard, inflexible surfaces like concrete increases the forces causing stress to the lumbar spine and should likewise be avoided.

Long-term prognosis
Unlike most stress fractures, spondylolysis (and spondylolisthesis) do not typically heal with time, although given adequate healing time, bone remodeling tends to repair lumbar fractures, particularly in less severe cases. Should rest and normal rehabilitation fail to restore mobility and should long-term pain persist, spinal surgery (in which the lumbar vertebrae are fused with the sacrum) may be necessary.

REHABILITATION EXERCISES

Barbell row

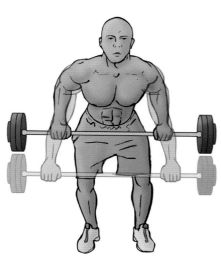

Stand with your knees slightly bent and lean forward at your waist. Hold on to a barbell with your hands placed slightly wider than your shoulders. Lift the bar by bringing it up towards your chest, then lower slowly and repeat.

Single arm dumbbell row

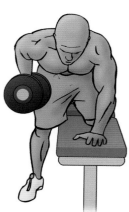

Place one knee and hand on a weight bench and grip a dumbbell with your other hand. Begin holding the dumbbell off the floor with your elbow bent at a 90-degree angle and your back almost parallel to the ground. Let the dumbbell slowly fall to the floor and lift it back up.

Pull-ups

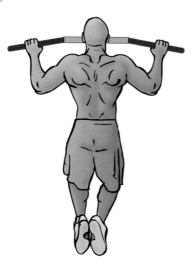

With both feet on the floor, reach up and grip a pull-up bar with your hands positioned slightly wider than your shoulders. Pull yourself up so that your chin rises above the bar. Slowly lower yourself to the start position without letting your feet touch the ground. Repeat.

Good mornings

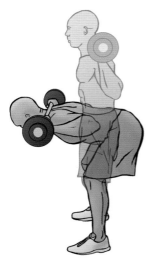

With your feet shoulder width apart and your knees slightly bent, position a barbell so it sits behind your neck. Slowly lean forward at your waist, keeping your back straight and your head up until your upper body is parallel to the ground. Then slowly raise the barbell back to your original position.

Alternate arm/leg raise

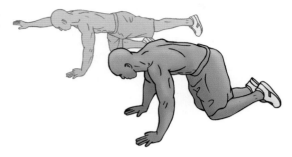

Kneel on the ground with your palms on the floor in front of you. Reach forward with one arm and backward with the opposite leg. Lower your arm and leg to the kneeling position and repeat with your other arm and leg.

Lying knee roll stretch

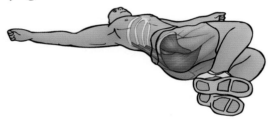

While lying on your back, bend your knees and let them fall to one side. Keep your arms out to the side and let your back and hips rotate with your knees.

Kneeling reach stretch

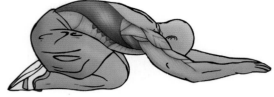

Kneel on the ground and reach forward with your hands. Let your head fall forward and push your buttocks towards your feet.

REHABILITATION EXERCISES

Sports Injuries of the Chest and Abdomen

ANATOMY AND PHYSIOLOGY

The ribcage protects the organs inside the chest (thoracic) cavity and is essential to the breathing mechanism. The muscles responsible for opening up the chest cavity, to allow air to enter the lungs, attach to the ribs. The ribs are more flexible than many other bones due to their cartilaginous attachments. Ribs attach to the sternum and/or costal margin at the front and articulate with the thoracic vertebrae at the back.

There are twelve pairs of ribs, comprising true, false and floating ribs. The first seven pairs (ribs 1–7) are known as true ribs, and attach via costal cartilage directly to the sternum. The next three pairs (ribs 8–10) are known as the false ribs, and attach to costal cartilage but not directly to the sternum. The final two pairs of ribs (ribs 11 and 12) are known as floating ribs, and lack attachment either to costal cartilage or to the sternum.

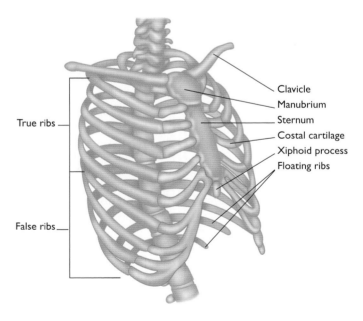

The ribs and sternum.

Breathing is a vital part of life and sport, and it is worth noting the main skeletal muscles involved.

The diaphragm is the main inspiratory muscle. Contraction of the muscle causes the dome of the diaphragm to descend, so enlarging the dimension of the thorax in all directions. The diaphragm contributes to spinal stability via an increase in intra-abdominal pressure, and with transversus abdominis, continually works to control trunk movement and enhance the breathing pattern during movement, particularly involving the extremities.

The outermost layer of the intercostal muscles is responsible for the lateral expansion of the chest and stabilization of the ribs during inspiration. Deep to them, the internal intercostals have an opposite action in forced expiration during exercise. The intercostals have a close anatomical connection with the internal and external oblique muscles.

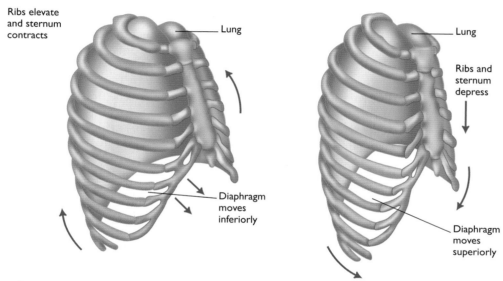

The mechanics of respiration.

The abdominal muscles are the main muscle group involved in forced expiration. These muscles alter the intra-abdominal pressure to assist the emptying of the lungs and transmit the pressure generated by the diaphragm. Intra-abdominal pressure is the pressure created within the trunk, in the closed cylinder of the diaphragm, pelvic floor and abdominal wall. Greater pressure adds stability to the trunk and pelvis.

The pelvic floor muscles are a collective group of muscles and soft tissue that makes up the base of the abdomino-pelvic cavity. These have a role in the maintenance of the intra-abdominal pressure and transference of the stability created by the respiratory process. Their main functions however are to support the internal pelvic organs and help to maintain continence.

Other muscle groups activated work with the main respiratory muscles but become activated when exercise becomes demanding. They are needed to stabilize parts of the body to enhance the respiratory action. The scalene muscles aid in deep inspiration by fixing the first and second ribs, and maintain them during expiration against the contraction of the abdominal muscles.

The sternocleidomastoid elevates the sternum and increases the forward and backward dimension of the chest during moderate to deep inspiration if the cervical spine is held stable. Serratus anterior assists in inspiration to laterally expand the rib cage, if the scapulae are stabilized.

The pectorals act in forced inspiration to raise the ribs, although the scapulae need to be stabilized by trapezius and serratus anterior to prevent scapular winging. Latissimus dorsi is involved in forced inspiration and expiration. Erector spinae helps in respiration by extending the thoracic spine and raising the rib cage. Quadratus lumborum stabilizes the twelfth rib to prevent elevation during respiration.

The anterior abdominal wall muscles run between the ribcage and the pelvis. They act to support the trunk, permit movement, hold the abdominal organs in place and support the lower back. There are three layers of muscle, with fibres running in the same direction as the corresponding three layers of muscle in the thoracic wall. The deepest layer consists of the transversus abdominis, whose fibres run approximately horizontally. The middle layer comprises the internal oblique, whose fibres are crossed by the outermost layer known as the external oblique, forming a pattern of fibres resembling an 'X'. Overlying these three layers is the rectus abdominis, which runs vertically, either side of the midline of the abdomen, and is associated with the 'six-pack' muscles seen in conditioned athletes.

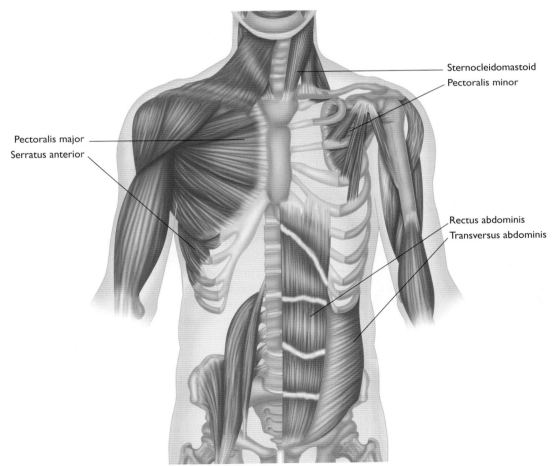

Muscles of the thoracic and abdominal region, anterior view.

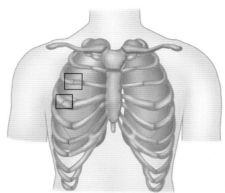

Broken (fractured) ribs.

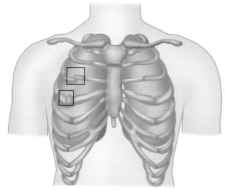

Flail chest.

BROKEN (FRACTURED) RIBS

Contact sports such as football and hockey, or sports that may result in falls or blunt trauma to the chest, have a higher incidence of rib fractures than other sports. Extreme sports, horseback riding, and martial arts are other examples of activities that may result in this injury. Pain and tenderness over the ribcage after blunt trauma or a fall, especially with difficulty breathing, should always be treated as potentially broken ribs and medical help sought. When the ribs or their cartilage components fracture or break, they weaken the support and protection of the chest cavity. This may interfere with the muscles' ability to open the chest cavity effectively to allow for adequate ventilation, which results in poor air intake and oxygen exchange. Any of the ribs may fracture, and often more than one rib is involved in the injury.

Cause of injury
Hard blow to the chest, side or back. Fall, landing on the chest, back or side. Forceful coughing – most common in people with impaired bone health, e.g. osteoporosis.

Signs and symptoms
Pain and tenderness over the fracture site, which may be noted also when pressing on the sternum or compressing the ribcage. Pain and difficulty breathing, especially on inhalation. Depending on the number of ribs involved, irregular movement of the chest during breathing may be noted, as well as some swelling.

Complications if left unattended
Fractured ribs that are left unattended will be painful and could lead to infections in the lungs due to shallow breathing. Reduced oxygen levels may result from the lower volume of air taken in. The bone ends may separate and cause damage to the delicate lung tissue underneath, causing a punctured lung or other damage; possibly even to the heart. Overall stability of the chest cavity will be affected also.

Immediate treatment
If a rib fracture is suspected, seek medical attention. Ice and anti-inflammatory medication may be used for pain relief. Compression may be used to stabilize the area until medical help is obtained, but should not be used long-term due to the limiting of deep, cleansing breaths needed for lung tissue health.

Rehabilitation and prevention
Rest is essential for recovery and repair of fractured ribs. It is important to take at least one deep, lung expanding breath each hour to ensure adequate lung tissue involvement and avoid infections in the lungs. Protecting the injured area until it is completely healed is important. Due to the inability to totally rest this area because of its constant movement during breathing, it takes longer to heal, usually 6–8 weeks. When returning to activity, this area should be padded and protected for an additional week or two.

Building muscle mass in the chest and back will help protect the ribs from injury. Using properly fitting and appropriate protective equipment will help to protect the ribs also. Avoiding trauma to the ribcage is the most important step in preventing rib fractures.

Long-term prognosis

Ribs usually heal completely if given adequate rest. The chances of breaking a rib are no greater after an initial break, if it is allowed to heal completely. The number of ribs involved in the injury may impact overall recovery time. If underlying tissue, such as the heart or lungs, is involved in the injury it may take much longer to heal completely and therefore may result in significant recovery time.

FLAIL CHEST

The ribs form a cage that protects the vital organs in thoracic cavity. When ribs are fractured in multiple places allowing portions to float free, flail chest may result. The chest wall is no longer one unit and the detached area may move separately from the rest of the chest wall. This is a serious condition due to the delicate nature of the underlying organs and the role of the ribs, and chest wall, in the process of breathing. This is a medical emergency and should be treated immediately. When a rib is broken in two or more places the integrity of the ribcage is compromised and the chest wall loses its support. This is especially true when more than one rib is involved in the injury. This may also occur when the costal cartilage is broken along with a fracture in the rib itself. The ability of the chest to expand and draw air into the lungs is affected and respirations become irregular and shallow. Paradoxical chest rise or uneven rise across the entire chest cavity often accompanies this injury, resulting in the chest collapsing during inhalation and expanding during exhalation.

Cause of injury

Blunt trauma to the ribcage. Fall or other direct blow to the chest, back or side. Crush injury to the thoracic area. Untreated rib fracture with additional trauma.

Signs and symptoms

Unequal or uneven chest rise. One area may seem to move independent of the rest of the chest and in opposition to normal respiratory rise. Pain and tenderness. Difficulty breathing. Bruising and possible swelling over the injured area. Instability in the chest wall over the fractured ribs.

Complications if left unattended

In flail chest, the broken ribs are floating free and may cause injury to the delicate lung and heart tissue immediately below. This could lead to a pneumothorax (air in the chest cavity causing partial or total collapse of the lung) or haemothorax (loss of blood into the pleural cavity around the lungs). Lung capacity and breathing are affected by the pain and instability associated with flail chest. The inability to properly ventilate the lungs could lead to hypoxia (a reduced concentration of oxygen in blood and tissues). The inability to fully inflate the lungs could lead to pneumonia and other respiratory complications.

Immediate treatment

This injury is a medical emergency due to the possible complications, and immediate medical help should be sought. Ice and anti-inflammatory or pain medication may be used for pain management. Compression of the injured area for stabilization may be used until medical help is obtained, but should not be used long-term due to the compromising of proper ventilation of the lungs.

Rehabilitation and prevention

Rest is the most important step in the recovery phase of this injury. Protecting the injured area is important as well. Return to activity should be slow and the injured area padded for additional protection. The muscles surrounding the injury site will require rehabilitation when the fractures have healed. This should be approached cautiously and gradually. Strengthening and building muscle mass around the ribcage will help protect it from injury. The thick muscles of the chest and back provide good protection. The side of the ribcage should be protected with protective gear. Avoiding trauma to the ribcage will also reduce the chances of this injury.

Long-term prognosis

Flail chest should recover fully with adequate rest and rehabilitation. In some cases surgical intervention may be required to stabilize the fractured ribs. When many ribs are involved, or multiple fractures are found in each rib, the recovery time will be increased. Damage to the underlying tissue, or to supportive tissues, may increase the overall healing time as well.

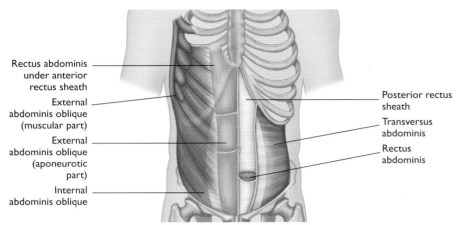

Rectus abdominis under anterior rectus sheath

External abdominis oblique (muscular part)

External abdominis oblique (aponeurotic part)

Internal abdominis oblique

Posterior rectus sheath

Transversus abdominis

Rectus abdominis

ABDOMINAL MUSCLE STRAIN

Strain to the abdominal muscles (also known as a pulled abdominal muscle) occurs from over-stretching and/or tearing of muscle fibres, a common injury in many sports. Such tearing tends to be mild but in severe cases the muscle can rupture.

Cause of injury
Muscle stretched too far. Muscle stretched while contracting. Sudden, violent movement of the trunk. Direct trauma.

Signs and symptoms
Abdominal pain at the injured muscle. Lower back pain. Muscle spasms, occasionally bruising.

Complications if left unattended
Muscle strains of the abdomen are common and usually resolve with rest, although continued vigorous exercise and inadequate healing time can lead to more serious damage to muscle and tendon, prolonged pain and interference with normal activity.

Immediate treatment
RICER regimen. Anti-inflammatory medication and analgesics.

Rehabilitation and prevention
Rest and adequate healing time are generally sufficient to relieve muscle strains of the abdomen and return the athlete to full capacity. Targeted exercises to strengthen the abdominal muscles, including slow repetition exercises for abdomen and spine, may then be undertaken. Attention to proper technique is critical in avoiding muscle strain injuries, as is thorough stretching prior to sports activity.

Long-term prognosis
Abdominal muscle strains broadly fall into three categories of severity, each requiring similar care but varying lengths of time for proper healing. Generally, a full recovery to normal sports activity can be expected. The condition occurring without serious complication does not require surgery.

REHABILITATION EXERCISES

Gym ball dumbbell press

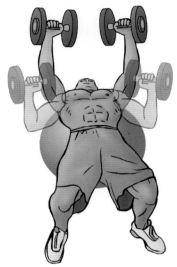

With both feet on the floor support your back with a gym ball. Start with your elbows bent and your hands holding a pair of dumbbells. Straighten your elbows by pushing the dumbbells directly upward. Lower the dumbbells to the starting position and repeat.

Flat dumbbell fly

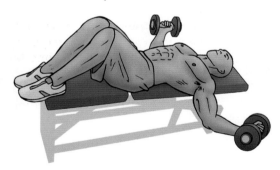

While lying on a weight bench grip a dumbbell in each hand. Start with your elbows slightly bent and your arms out to the side. Keeping a slight bend in your elbows raise the dumbbells up until they meet above your chest. Slowly lower the dumbbells to the start position and repeat.

Gym ball crunch

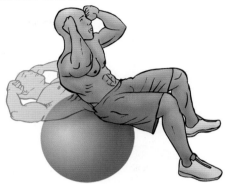

Sit upright on a gym ball with both feet on the ground. Rest your hands gently against the side of your head and slowly lower your upper body down towards the gym ball. Raise your upper body back to the start position and repeat.

Weighted seated twist

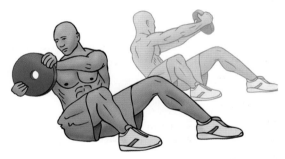

Sit on the ground with your feet in front of you and let your upper body lean back slightly until your body position resembles a 'V'. Grip a plate out in front of your chest while keeping your elbows slightly bent. Rotate your upper body moving the plate from side to side.

Hanging leg raise

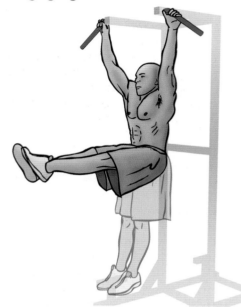

With your arms supporting you, let your legs fall with your toes hanging off the ground. Raise your legs until they are parallel to the ground. Let them fall slowly back to the start position and repeat.

Door frame chest stretch

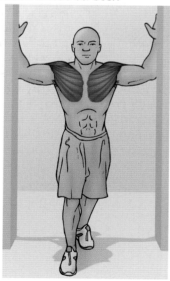

Stand in a doorway with your hands resting on both sides of the frame at about head level. Keeping your hands and feet outside the door, let your upper body's weight slowly fall forward through the doorway.

Back arch stomach stretch

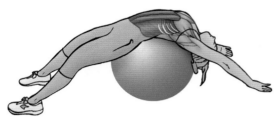

With both feet on the ground, push back against a gym ball until your shoulders and neck are not supported by it. Raise your arms above your head and reach as far back toward the ground as you can.

Lateral side stretch

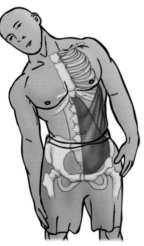

Stand with your feet about shoulder width apart and look forward. Keep your body upright and slowly bend to the left or right. Reach down your leg with your hand and do not bend forward.

Sports Injuries of the Hips, Pelvis and Groin

ANATOMY AND PHYSIOLOGY

The pelvic girdle (or hip girdle) consists of two pelvic or coxal bones. It provides a strong and stable support for the vertebral column and pelvic organs, and connects the vertebral column with the lower limbs. The pelvic bones unite with one another in the front (anteriorly) at the pubic symphysis, a stable joint reinforced by strong ligaments and a fibrocartilage disc. With the sacrum and coccyx, the two pelvic bones form a basin-like structure called the pelvis. At birth, each coxal bone consists of three separate bones: the ilium, the ischium and the pubis. These bones eventually fuse and the area where they join is a deep hemispherical socket called the acetabulum which articulates with the head of the femur. Although the pelvic bone is one bone it is commonly discussed in terms of its three portions.

The ilium is a large, flaring bone that forms the largest and most superior portion of the pelvic bone. The iliac crests are felt when you rest your hands on your hips. Each crest terminates in the front at the anterior superior iliac spine (ASIS) and at the back as the posterior superior iliac spine (PSIS) The PSIS is difficult to palpate but its position is revealed by a skin dimple in the sacral region, level approximately to the second sacral foramen.

The ischium is the inferior, posterior part of the pelvic bone. It is roughly arch-shaped. At the bottom of the ischium are the roughened and thickened ischial tuberosities (sometimes called the 'sit-bones' because when we sit our weight is borne entirely by the ischial tuberosities). The pubis is the anterior and inferior part of the pelvic bone and is made up of two bony processes or rami.

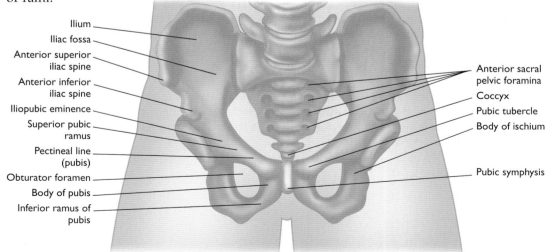

Bones of the pelvic girdle, anterior view.

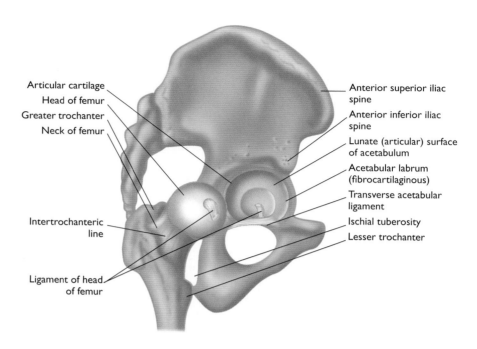

Articular cartilage
Head of femur
Greater trochanter
Neck of femur
Intertrochanteric line
Ligament of head of femur

Anterior superior iliac spine
Anterior inferior iliac spine
Lunate (articular) surface of acetabulum
Acetabular labrum (fibrocartilaginous)
Transverse acetabular ligament
Ischial tuberosity
Lesser trochanter

The hip joint, right leg, lateral view.

The most important hip flexor muscles are iliopsoas (iliacus and psoas major) and rectus femoris. Their function is to pull the femur up toward the abdomen, or conversely to pull the abdomen down toward the legs, as in a sit-up. Runners, cyclists, soccer players, hikers, and people involved in jumping activities where the legs are lifted raised are all at risk of hip flexor strains.

The groin area covers the inner thigh and the junction between the torso and legs. The muscles of the groin include the pectineus, adductor brevis, adductor longus, gracilis and adductor magnus. These muscles are responsible for pulling the leg in toward the midline of the body and attach at the pelvis and the femur, some up high and others closer to the knee.

The piriformis muscle is a small, triangular muscle that originates at the internal surface of the sacrum and inserts onto the greater trochanter of the femur. Piriformis leaves the pelvis by passing through the greater sciatic foramen. The muscle assists in laterally rotating the hip joint, abducting the thigh when the hip is flexed, and helps to hold the head of the femur in the acetabulum.

Iliopsoas is actually made of two muscles: the iliacus, which originates at the hip bone, and psoas major which originates at the lumbar spine. Both muscles share their insertion via a common tendon at the top of the femur. The iliopsoas muscle is the main flexor of the hip joint.

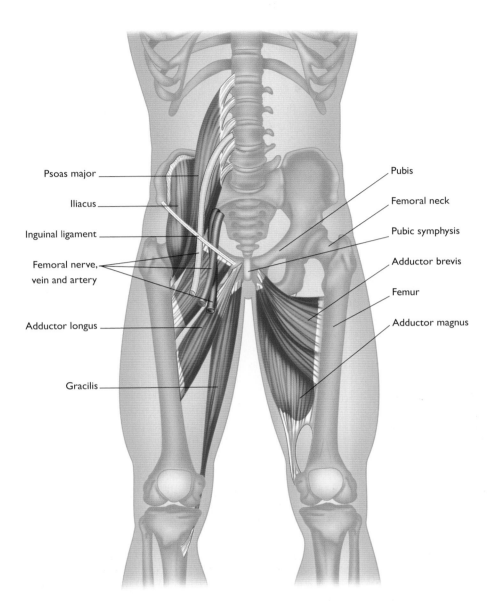

Psoas major

Iliacus

Inguinal ligament

Femoral nerve, vein and artery

Adductor longus

Gracilis

Pubis

Femoral neck

Pubic symphysis

Adductor brevis

Femur

Adductor magnus

The iliopsoas, adductors and pelvic region, anterior view.

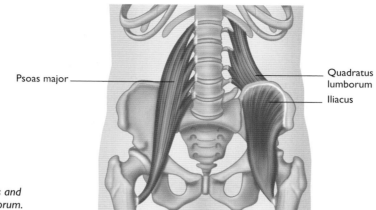

Deep hip flexors and quadratus lumborum.

HIP FLEXOR STRAIN

Hip flexors are located on the front of the hip and lift the thigh up or bend the waist forward or down when the limbs are fixed. These muscles are used a lot in cycling, running, kicking and jumping activities. When a new load is placed on the muscle or repetitive stresses are encountered without rest, the muscle may stretch or tear.

Cause of injury
Repetitive stress on the hip flexor muscles without adequate time for recovery. Excessive stress placed on the muscles without appropriate strengthening and warm-up. Improper form when running, cycling or other activities. Forceful hyperextension of the leg at the hip.

Signs and symptoms
Pain in the upper groin area over the anterior portion of the hip. Pain with movement of the leg at the hip. Inflammation and tenderness over the hip flexor.

Complications if left unattended
Hip flexor strains left untreated can become chronic and lead to inflexible muscles that could lead to other injuries. The muscle could also continue to tear, eventually leading to a complete rupture from the attachment.

Immediate treatment
Cessation of activities that aggravate the hip flexors. Ice for the first 48–72 hours. Anti-inflammatory medication. Then heat and massage to promote blood flow and healing.

Rehabilitation and prevention
Conditioning is the key to rehabilitation and prevention of hip flexor strains. Muscles that are strong and flexible are much more resilient. Stretching the hip flexors, abdominals, lower back, quadriceps and hamstrings helps to lower the stress load placed on the hip flexors. Strengthening of iliopsoas and the other muscles of the hip, quadriceps, lower back and abdomen will help to prepare the hip flexors for unexpected stresses.

Long-term prognosis
Although the potential for chronic pain and inflexibility exists, hip flexor strains usually recover fully when given adequate rest and active recovery using stretching and strengthening exercises.

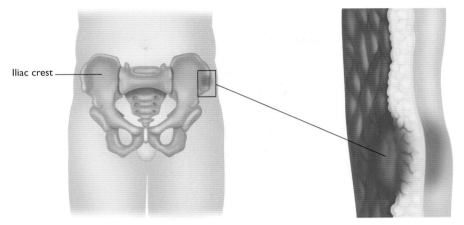

Iliac crest

HIP POINTER

Hip pointer usually refers to a deep bruise of the iliac crest and the muscles that cover it. It is often caused by a direct blow. Hip pointers are most commonly associated with football but may be seen in any contact sport.

A hip pointer is usually a bruise of the muscle or bone but can be as severe as a chip or fracture. The iliac crest (felt when you rest your hands on your hips) is the area of bone involved and the muscles that attach to it include the hip flexors, the abdominals and the gluteal muscles responsible for the rotation of the hips. Because these muscles are injured at their attachments any movement involving these muscles will be painful.

Cause of injury
Direct impact to the hip.

Signs and symptoms
Pain and tenderness over the iliac crest. Pain with movement of the hip and sometimes with weightbearing (due to the muscle involvement). Local inflammation, bruising and swelling.

Complications if left unattended
Left unattended, the pain and inflammation can lead to improper gait and become chronic. If the bone is chipped or fractured, failure to treat can lead to improper healing and future injuries to the site.

Immediate treatment
Cessation of the activity. Ice the area immediately. X-ray for possible fracture or bone chips.

Rehabilitation and prevention
Use of proper protective equipment during activities and strengthening the supporting muscles around the hip for added padding and protection. Unfortunately there is not a lot that can be done to prevent falling or contact with the hip area.

Rehabilitation includes rest until the pain subsides, then gradual reintroduction to the activity. Any activities causing pain should be discontinued until the area is pain free.

Long-term prognosis
Hip pointers seldom cause long-term disability and most athletes can return to full function after treatment and a rehabilitation period. Surgery is seldom required except in severe fracture cases.

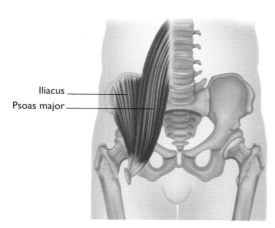

Iliacus

Psoas major

AVULSION FRACTURE

An avulsion fracture occurs when a tendon or ligament pulls away from the bone at its attachment, pulling a piece of the bone away with it. This usually results from a forceful twisting muscular contraction, or powerful hyperextension or hyperflexion. This injury is more prevalent in children than in adults. The tendon or ligament tends to tear before the bone is involved in adults, but the softer bones tend to become involved in children. Avulsion fractures are commonly seen in boys aged between 13 and 17, although the ligament-bone junction is a common site of injury in middle-aged people.

Although any tendon or ligament in the body can be involved in an avulsion fracture, it is more common in those around the pelvis. Avulsion fractures most commonly occur at apophyses, sites where a major tendon attaches onto a growing bony prominence. In children, the growth plate is a weaker site where the bone is still forming, and is an area where avulsion fractures often occur. The anterior superior iliac spine (ASIS), anterior inferior iliac spine (AIIS) and the ischial tuberosity are the bony prominences most commonly involved. The corresponding muscles affected are sartorius, rectus femoris and the hamstrings (see page 178) respectively.

Cause of injury

Forceful twisting, extending or flexing causing extra stress on the ligaments or tendons. Direct impact on a joint causing forceful stretching of the ligaments.

Signs and symptoms

Pain, swelling and tenderness at the injury site. Sudden localized pain that may radiate down the muscle.

Complications if left unattended

Left untreated an avulsion fracture will lead to long-term disability in the muscles and joints involved. Incomplete or incorrect healing may lead to injuries to other muscles.

Immediate treatment

RICER regimen. Immobilization of the joint involved. Anti-inflammatory medication. Seek immediate medical help.

Rehabilitation and prevention

Initial rest for the injured muscles and joints followed by strengthening of the muscles and supporting ligaments will help rehabilitate and prevent future fractures. Gradual re-entry into full activity is important to prevent re-injuring the weakened area.

Long-term prognosis

With proper treatment most simple avulsion fractures will heal completely with no limitations. In rare cases surgery may be needed to repair the avulsed bone, especially in children when the avulsion involves a growth plate.

GROIN STRAIN

As with any strain, groin strain (also known as rider's strain) is a stretch or tear of any or all of the adductor muscles of the inner thigh or their tendons. Soccer, hockey and other sports that require pivoting and quick direction changes are the most common activities for groin pulls. These injuries range from simple stretching of the muscles to more severe tearing of the fibres. As with other strains it is graded 1 through to 3 with 3 being the most severe tear.

Due to this location and function, athletes involved in sports where the leg is moved forcefully inward or outward are more susceptible to this injury. Damage is usually to the musculo-tendinous junction, about 5 cm from the pubis.

Cause of injury
Forceful stretching of the adductor muscles of the hip. Forceful contraction of the adductor muscles.

Signs and symptoms
Grade 1: Mild pain. Stiffness in the adductor muscles but little or no effect on athletic performance.
Grade 2: More painful. Some swelling, tenderness, limited range of motion, pain when walking or jogging.
Grade 3: Very painful. Significant swelling, pain with weight bearing, sometimes pain at rest or at night.

Complications if left unattended
Untreated groin strains can lead to an awkward gait and chronic pain that could lead to injuries in other areas. A minor muscle tear could become more severe and eventually tear completely.

Immediate treatment
RICER. Anti-inflammatory medication. For a Grade 3 strain it may be necessary to seek a medical evaluation.

Rehabilitation and prevention
After initial treatment, minor strains will respond to a gradual stretching and strengthening programme. More serious strains will require additional rest and a slow entry back into activities with extra warm-up activities before each session.

Prevention of groin strains requires warming-up properly before activities, stretching for good flexibility in the adductors and strengthening of the abductor muscles, adductor muscles, abdominals and hip flexors for good muscular balance.

Long-term prognosis
Most groin strains will heal with no lasting effects. Only the most severe strains, with complete tears, require surgical correction.

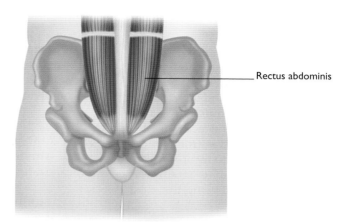

Rectus abdominis

OSTEITIS PUBIS

Osteitis pubis is an inflammation of the pubic symphysis and the surrounding muscles. This is a chronic problem that often results from a muscle imbalance, repetitive stresses or an untreated injury to the bones or musculature of the area. Soccer players, hockey players, sprinters and other athletes who are involved in running, kicking or rapid lateral movements are more susceptible to this type of injury.

The pubic symphysis with its fibrocartilage disc is involved in this injury. No instability of the pubic symphysis occurs, but there is tenderness over the area. The adductor muscles and hip flexors are also involved. Repetitive stresses on this area or a change in the angle of stress, from a major trauma, can lead to a change in the structure of the pubic symphysis. This causes a shift in the pull of the muscles attached there.

Cause of injury

Repetitive stresses on the pubic symphysis from running, kicking, etc. Unresolved trauma to this area resulting in abnormal forces on the pubic symphysis.

Signs and symptoms

Adductor or lower abdominal pain that localizes to the pubic area. Pain increases with running, kicking or pushing off to change direction.

Complications if left unattended

Untreated osteitis pubis will lead to increased pain and disability. The increased pain may lead to awkward form during certain activities which could lead to other injuries.

Immediate treatment

Ice and rest from aggravating activities. Anti-inflammatory medication.

Rehabilitation and prevention

Restoring flexibility to the entire hip girdle when the pain subsides. Gradual re-introduction to athletic activity. Stop an activity if it causes pain. Strengthening the adductor muscles and the hip flexors helps prepare this area to handle the stresses more efficiently. Proper warm-up techniques before running, kicking or other direct impact activities are also important.

Long-term prognosis

When treated properly there are seldom any long-term effects. Full range of motion and strength should return. If pain and limited mobility linger the injury should be re-evaluated.

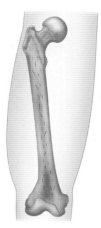

STRESS FRACTURE

Repetitive stress or unnatural stress placed on the surface of bone, often from muscle fatigue, can lead to stress fractures. Running, jumping and other high-impact activities can cause small cracks or fractures along a bone. Stress fractures may occur in any bone subjected to repetitive stress or impact.

Stress fractures are most commonly found in the bones of the foot, lower leg and hip. When a muscle becomes fatigued and can no longer absorb the shock of impact, that stress gets transferred to the bone. Over time that stress will cause small cracks in the bone. Fatigue in certain muscles may also create strength imbalances that put an unnatural stress on the bone causing small fractures. Stress fractures to the pubis, femoral neck and proximal third of the femur are seen in individuals who perform aerobic dance activities or extensive jogging.

Cause of injury
Repetitive stress from impact activities. Unnatural stress on a bone from different running surfaces. Strength imbalances causing unusual stress.

Signs and symptoms
Generalized area of pain. Pain on weightbearing. When running, the pain is severe in the beginning, with no or moderate pain in the middle, and severe pain returning at the end of or after the run.

Complications if left unattended
When left unattended a stress fracture may develop into a more serious complete fracture. The pain and natural guarding of the injured area can lead to injury in other areas.

Immediate treatment
Rest is the most important treatment. Anti-inflammatory medication.

Rehabilitation and prevention
When recovering from a stress fracture it is important to start activity slowly. It may take 4–8 weeks for a fracture to completely heal. During that time it is important to identify training problems that may have caused the stress fracture originally. It is also important during this time to keep up general conditioning using activities that do not require excessive impact on the affected area.

To prevent stress fractures, it is important to warm-up properly and use proper equipment (avoid using worn out running shoes, etc.). Increase exercise intensity slowly and eat plenty of calcium-rich foods to support bone repair and growth.

Long-term prognosis
With proper treatment and rehabilitation most stress fractures heal completely with no future concerns. A rare few may require surgical pinning to strengthen the fracture area.

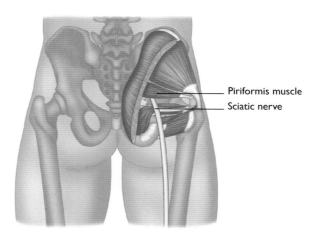

Piriformis muscle
Sciatic nerve

PIRIFORMIS SYNDROME

Piriformis syndrome is a result of impingement of the sciatic nerve by the piriformis muscle. Incorrect form or improper gait often leads to tightness and inflexibility in piriformis. The condition occurs more frequently in women than men (6:1). When piriformis becomes tight it puts pressure on the underlying nerve, causing pain similar to sciatica. The pain usually starts in the mid-gluteal region and radiates down the back of the thigh.

Cause of injury

Incorrect form or gait while walking or jogging. Weak gluteal muscles and/or tight adductor muscles.

Signs and symptoms

Pain along the sciatic nerve. Pain when climbing stairs or walking up an incline. Increased pain after prolonged sitting.

Complications if left unattended

Chronic pain will result if left untreated. The tight muscle could also become irritated causing stress on the tendons and points of attachment.

Immediate treatment

RICER. Anti-inflammatory medication. Then heat and massage to promote blood flow and healing.

Rehabilitation and prevention

During rehabilitation a gradual return to activity and continued stretching of the hip muscles is essential. Start with lower exercise intensity or duration. Identifying the factors that caused the problem is also important. Strengthening the gluteal muscles and increasing the flexibility of the adductors will help to alleviate some of the stress and prevent the piriformis from becoming tight. Maintaining a good stretching regimen to keep the piriformis muscle flexible will help, while dealing with the other issues.

Long-term prognosis

Piriformis syndrome seldom results in long-term problems when treated properly. Rarely, a corticosteroid injection or other invasive method may be required to alleviate symptoms.

ILIOPSOAS TENDINITIS

Inflammation of the iliopsoas tendon and is usually caused by overuse or incorrect use of equipment. The iliopsoas muscle and tendon can become inflamed through repetitive hip flexion, such as is involved in running, jumping and even weight training that involves a lot of bending and squatting. Occasionally the underlying bursa will also become inflamed.

Cause of injury
Repetitive hip flexion such as running, jumping and kicking. Untreated trauma to the iliopsoas muscle.

Signs and symptoms
Pain with hip movement. Tenderness over the upper groin. Onset is gradual and pain worsens with activity.

Complications if left unattended
Tendinitis can eventually lead to a muscle tear if left untreated and the activity that caused it continues. Bursitis is also another problem that may develop from unattended tendinitis.

Immediate treatment
RICER. Anti-inflammatory medication. Then heat and massage to promote blood flow and healing.

Rehabilitation and prevention
Once most of the pain has been managed it is important to start working on the strength and flexibility in the affected muscle. Increasing the flexibility in the muscles responsible for hip extension (gluteus maximus and the hamstrings) will speed recovery and reduce the chance of recurrence. Proper warm-up before activity and developing a strength balance between hip flexors and extensors will also help prevent this injury.

Long-term prognosis
Iliopsoas tendinitis seldom needs more than the initial treatment and rehabilitation to recover fully. If pain persists or becomes more severe it may be necessary to consult a physician.

TENDINITIS OF THE ADDUCTOR MUSCLES

Inflammation in the adductor muscle tendons or tendon sheaths due to overuse can cause pain in the groin area. Sprinting, football, hurdling and horse riding can all cause overuse in these muscles. Unresolved injuries such as groin strain can also lead to tendinitis.

The adductor muscles include the pectineus, adductor longus, adductor brevis, gracilis and adductor magnus and the tendons any of these may become inflamed. The pain is similar to a groin strain but onset is gradual and chronic in nature.

Cause of injury
Repetitive stress to the adductor muscles. Previous injury such as groin strain. Tight gluteal muscles.

Signs and symptoms
Pain in the groin area. Pain when bringing the legs together against resistance. Pain when running, especially sprinting.

Complications if left unattended
If left unattended, tendinitis of the adductor muscles can lead to imbalance and injury to the other muscles of the hip joint. It can also result in a tear of one or more of the adductor muscles.

Immediate treatment
Ice and rest from activities that cause pain. Anti-inflammatory medication. Then heat and massage to promote blood flow and healing.

Rehabilitation and prevention
Rehabilitation for tendinitis of the adductors starts with gradual reintroduction into activity with stretching and strengthening exercises for the affected muscles. Use heat packs on the affected area before exercise at first, then continue with good warm-up activities to make sure the muscles are ready for activity. Strengthening the adductors and stretching the opposing abductors will help prevent this injury from recurring. Rehabilitating all groin pulls and other hip injuries completely will also prevent problems with the adductors.

Long-term prognosis
Long-term problems are seldom seen with tendinitis of the adductor muscles after treatment. If pain and limited mobility in the hip persists, additional help may be required from a sports medicine specialist.

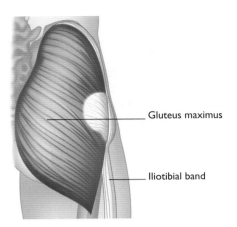

Gluteus maximus

Iliotibial band

SNAPPING HIP SYNDROME

Snapping hip syndrome is a condition where a snapping or popping sensation is felt in the hip with hip flexion and extension. It is most commonly caused by a tendon snapping over a bony prominence. This syndrome may present with or without pain and is particularly prevalent in dancers.

External snapping hip syndrome can be the result of a tight 'Iliotibial band' (ITB) or gluteus maximus tendon snapping over the greater trochanter of the femur. When landing from a jump, running, climbing or squatting these tendons are forced over the bony prominence of the greater trochanter. This can cause inflammation of the muscle and tendon.

Internal snapping syndrome may be caused by the iliopsoas tendon snapping over the iliopectineal eminence of the hip. In more rare cases, tearing of the cartilage (labral tears) of the hip joint may cause snapping as well.

Cause of injury

Tight ITB or gluteal muscles. Tight iliopsoas muscle. Labral tear.

Signs and symptoms

Snapping sensation in the hip. May or may not present with pain (more commonly reported as discomfort).

Complications if left unattended

Snapping hip syndrome can lead to irritation and possible bursitis if left untreated. The inflamed muscle becomes tight and can cause stress on other muscles as well.

Immediate treatment

RICER programme. Anti-inflammatory medication.

Rehabilitation and prevention

Rehabilitation starts with stretching and strengthening the muscles of the hip. A balance in strength and flexibility of all the muscles will help prevent snapping hip syndrome. Proper warm-up of the hip muscles is important before beginning any activity that involves flexion or extension to make sure the muscles are adequately prepared. It is also important to maintain fitness levels while resting, using activities that do not aggravate the affected area.

Long-term prognosis

Snapping hip syndrome seldom requires more than the initial treatment and rehabilitation to recover fully. In very rare cases surgical intervention may be required to correct the problem.

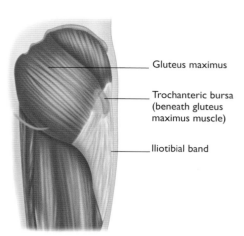

Gluteus maximus

Trochanteric bursa
(beneath gluteus
maximus muscle)

Iliotibial band

TROCHANTERIC BURSITIS

Trochanteric bursitis commonly results when the bursa over the greater trochanter of the femur is irritated by repetitive stresses encountered during running activities. The greater trochanter is the bony prominence on the upper lateral portion of the femur to which many muscles of the hip and thigh attach. The trochanteric bursa lies between gluteus maximus and the posterolateral surface of the greater trochanter. Several other muscles cross this region and because they are generally rubbing across the bone the bursa can become inflamed. The greater trochanter is near the surface and is susceptible to impact injuries. Trochanteric bursitis may also be caused by tension in the iliotibial band (ITB).

Cause of injury

Repetitive activities involving the hip such as running. Impact or other trauma to the bursa over the greater trochanter. Limited ITB movement.

Signs and symptoms

Tenderness over the bony prominence of the upper thigh/hip. Swelling over the bursa. Pain when flexing or extending the hip.

Complications if left unattended

If left unattended this injury can cause chronic pain. The bursa may rupture with continued irritation of an already inflamed area.

Immediate treatment

Rest from aggravating activities. Ice. Anti-inflammatory medication.

Rehabilitation and prevention

Rest from activities that aggravate the bursa is the first step to reducing pain and inflammation. After rest a gradual return to sport is advised. Stop any activities that cause a recurrence of the pain. Creating a balance of strength and flexibility in all the muscles of the hip will help prevent trochanteric bursitis. Warming up the muscles of the hip properly before activity is also important.

Long-term prognosis

Bursitis generally does not cause any long-term disability when treatment and rehabilitation programmes are followed. Surgery is only indicated in very extreme cases.

REHABILITATION EXERCISES

Lunge

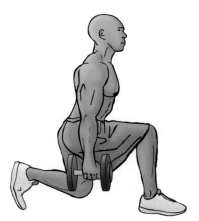

With a dumbbell in each hand resting at your sides, step forward with one foot while letting your opposite knee fall almost to the ground. Push upward, returning to the start position, then step forward with your other foot letting your other knee do the same.

Body weight squat

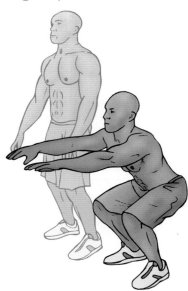

With your feet shoulder width apart, reach your hands out in front of you and bend your knees like you are about to sit in a chair. Slowly return to standing and repeat.

Single-legged gluteal raise hold

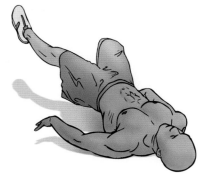

Lie on your back with your arms at your sides. Keep one leg straight and bring the other foot up towards your backside. Raise your backside off the ground, hold for a second and then lower again. Repeat with your other leg.

Side step lunge

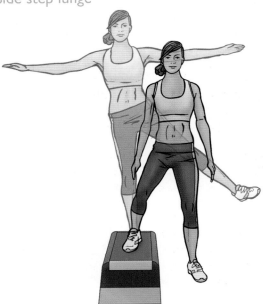

With one foot elevated on a support, bring your arms out from your sides and lift your other leg up and away from your body to the side.

Hanging knee raise

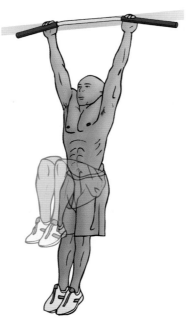

While hanging on a bar with your feet off the ground, lift and bend your knees while keeping your arms straight. Bring them as close to your chest as possible. Slowly lower to the start position and repeat.

Leg out adductor stretch

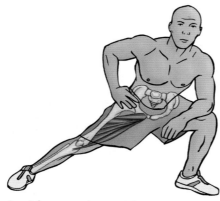

Stand with your feet wide apart. Keep one leg straight and toes facing forward while bending the other leg and turning your toes out to the side. Lower your groin toward the ground and rest your hands on the bent knee or the ground.

Knee up rotation stretch

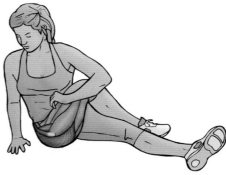

Sit with one leg straight and the other leg crossed over your knee. Turn your shoulders and put your arm onto your raised knee to help rotate your shoulders and back.

Lying foot over knee

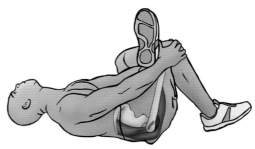

Lie on your back and slightly bend one leg. Raise your other foot up onto your bent leg and rest it on your thigh. Then reach forward holding on to your knee and pull your bent leg toward you.

13 Sports Injuries of the Hamstrings and Quadriceps

ANATOMY AND PHYSIOLOGY

The femur, or thigh bone, is the heaviest, longest and strongest bone in the body. Its proximal end has a ball-like head that articulates with the pelvic bone in the acetabulum and forms the hip joint. Distally the lateral and medial condyles articulate with the tibia to form the knee joint. The quadriceps, hamstrings, adductor and abductor muscles all have attachments on the femur.

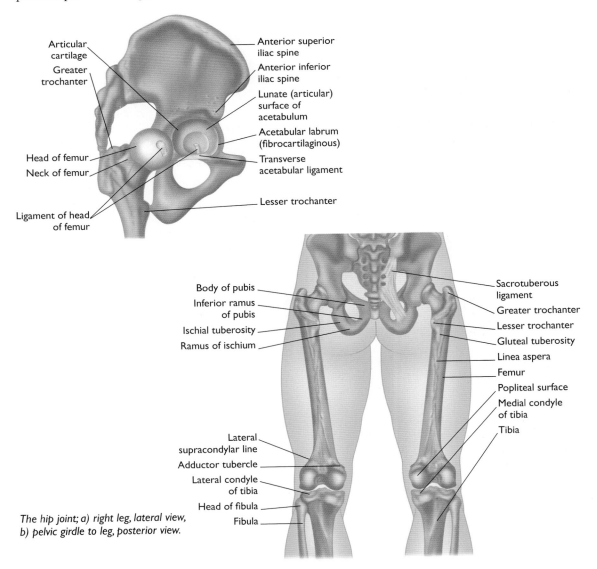

The hip joint; a) right leg, lateral view,
b) pelvic girdle to leg, posterior view.

The hamstrings are a group of three muscles that work together to extend (straighten) the hip and flex (bend) the knee. During running the hamstrings slow down the leg at the end of its forward swing and prevent the trunk from flexing at the hip joint. The three muscles are: biceps femoris, semitendinosus and semimembranosus.

The quadriceps group is composed of four muscles: vastus lateralis, vastus medialis, vastus intermedius and rectus femoris. The quadriceps tendon attaches to and surrounds the patella (kneecap), becoming the patellar (tendon) ligament below this and inserting on the anterior surface of the tibia. The patella moves up and down in the groove at the front of the femur as the knee flexes and extends which results in the tendon passing over this bone as well.

The iliotibial band (ITB) is a non-elastic collagen cord stretching from the lateral pelvis to below the knee. It is attached to the iliac crest at the top, blends with the tensor fasciae latae (TFL) and gluteus maximus muscles, and descends to attach to Gerdy's tubercle on the lateral proximal tibia. The deep fibres attach to the linea aspera of the femur on the posterolateral thigh. TFL flexes, abducts and medially rotates the hip joint, and stabilizes the knee.

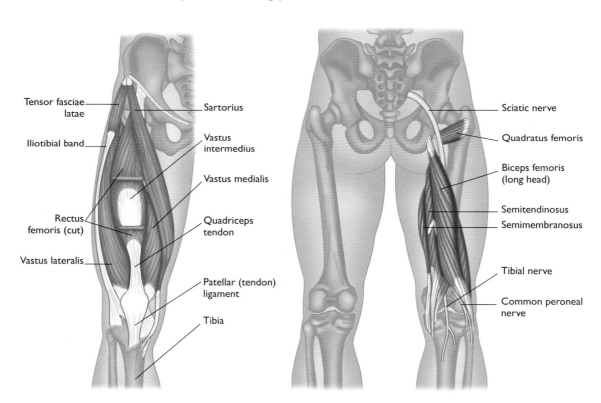

The quadriceps.   *The hamstrings.*

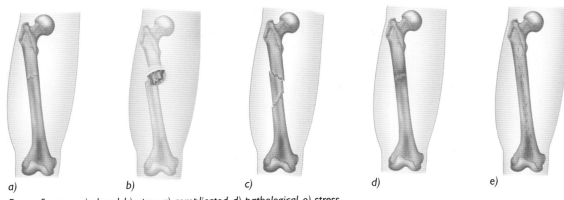

Femur fracture: a) closed, b) open, c) complicated, d) pathological, e) stress.

FEMUR FRACTURE

It takes tremendous force to fracture the femur due to its strength and the supporting musculature. Football, hockey and other high-impact sports are often associated with femoral fractures. The femur is more likely to fracture at the femoral neck, as it is smaller in diameter and is composed of cancellous bone which has a relatively low density. Femoral neck fractures usually involve a hard impact or excessive landing force from a high fall. The femur may also fracture along the shaft, which is usually caused by tremendous impact from a road traffic accident or shearing force across the bone.

Cause of injury

High-impact force across the femur, such as a car accident or aggressive tackle in football. High-impact force directed through the femur such as from landing from a high fall. Direct impact to the upper portion of the hip.

Signs and symptoms

Severe pain. Deformity and possible shortening of leg length. Swelling and discolouration. Inability to move the leg or bear weight.

Complications if left unattended

Permanent disability will result if this injury is left untreated. Blood loss due to internal injuries to the muscles and arteries could lead to shock and death.

Immediate treatment

Ice and immobilization. Seek immediate medical help.

Rehabilitation and prevention

Femoral fractures require extensive rehabilitation due to the time needed for healing and the musculature involved. The bone may require surgical repair with a plate, rod or pins, which increases the rehabilitation time. Rehabilitation will usually involve a physical therapist working on range of motion and strengthening the muscles.

Prevention of femoral fracture requires common sense safety precautions and/or avoidance of activities that might result in high-impact blows to the femur. Strengthening the muscles of the quadriceps, hamstrings, adductors and abductors will also provide extra protection for the femur.

Long-term prognosis

With immediate treatment and repair of the femur along with rehabilitation to strengthen the supporting muscles, there should be no long-term limitations. Full recovery may take up to nine months.

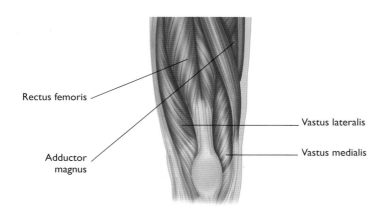

Rectus femoris

Vastus lateralis

Vastus medialis

Adductor magnus

QUADRICEPS STRAIN

A forceful stretch or tear of the muscle or tendon in a weightbearing muscle such as the quadriceps is painful and difficult to rest. The quadriceps are involved in supporting the hip and knee to hold the weight of the. A quadriceps strain can result from a forceful contraction of the quadriceps or unusual stress placed on the muscles. As with other strains it is graded 1 through 3, with 3 being the most severe tear.

A strain may occur in any of the quadriceps muscles but the rectus femoris is most commonly injured. The force generated in activities such as sprinting, jumping and weight training may cause microtears in the muscle. When the muscle is stretched forcefully under a load as in high-impact sports like football and hockey it may also pull away from the muscle–tendon junction or bony attachment or tear completely.

Cause of injury

Forceful contraction or stretch of the quadriceps.

Signs and symptoms

Grade 1: Mildly tender and painful. Little or no swelling. Full muscular strength.
Grade 2: More marked pain and tenderness. Moderate swelling and possible bruising. Noticeable loss of strength.
Grade 3 (full tear): Extreme pain. Deformity, swelling and bruising. Inability to contract the muscle.

Complications if left unattended

A grade 1 or 2 tear left unattended can continue to tear and become worse. A grade 3 tear left untreated can result in loss of mobility and a severe loss of flexibility in the muscle.

Immediate treatment

RICER regimen. Anti-inflammatory medication. Immobilization in severe cases. Then heat and massage to promote blood flow and healing.

Rehabilitation and prevention

After the required rest period, activities should be resumed cautiously. Avoid activities that cause pain. Stretching and strengthening of the quadriceps will be necessary. Ensuring a balance of strength between the quadriceps and hamstrings is important to prevent a strain. Proper warm-up techniques must be observed to prevent strains and gradually increasing intensity will help as well.

Long-term prognosis

Quadriceps strains seldom result in long-term pain or disability. Surgery is only needed in rare cases where a complete tear does not respond to immobilization and rest.

HAMSTRING STRAIN

A hamstring strain or 'pull' is a stretch or tear of the hamstring muscles or tendons. This is a very common injury, especially in activities that involve sprinting or explosive accelerations. A common cause of a hamstring strain is muscle imbalance between the hamstring and quadriceps, with the quadriceps being much stronger.

Any of the hamstring muscles can be strained. Commonly minor tears happen in the belly of the biceps femoris muscle closest to the knee. Complete tears or ruptures usually pull away from this attachment as well. Excessive force against the muscles, especially during eccentric contraction (when the muscle is contracting and lengthening against force) can cause stretching, minor tears or even complete rupture.

Cause of injury
Strength imbalance between the hamstrings and quadriceps. Forceful stretching of the muscle, especially during contraction. Excessive overload on the muscle.

Signs and symptoms
Grade 1: Mildly tender and painful. Little or no swelling. Full muscular strength.
Grade 2: More marked pain and tenderness. Moderate swelling and possible bruising. Gait affected - limping.
Grade 3 (full tear): Extreme pain. Marked swelling and bruising. Inability to bear weight.

Complications if left unattended
Pain and tightness in the hamstring muscles will get worse without treatment. Tightness in the hamstrings can lead to lower back and hip problems. Untreated strains can progress to a full rupture.

Immediate treatment
Grade 1: Ice. Anti-inflammatory medication.
Grades 2 and 3: RICER. Anti-inflammatory medication. Seek medical help if a complete rupture is suspected or if the patient is unable to walk unaided. Then heat and massage to promote blood flow and healing.

Rehabilitation and prevention
Stretching after the initial pain subsides will help speed recovery and prevent future recurrences. Strengthening the hamstrings to balance them with the quadriceps is also important. When re-entering activity, proper warm-up must be stressed and a gradual increase in intensity is important.

Long-term prognosis
Hamstring strains that are rehabilitated fully seldom leave any lingering effects. Complete ruptures may require surgery to repair and long-term rehabilitation.

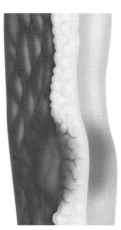

THIGH BRUISE

A thigh contusion is a deep bruise to the muscles of the quadriceps or hamstrings near the femur. The bruising causes pain and limited flexibility in the muscle. An impact to any of the hamstring or quadriceps muscles squeezes the muscle between the impacting force and the underlying bone. This causes bleeding in the muscle, inflammation and eventually the formation of scar tissue which reduces muscle function. Swelling and bruising from inflammation and bleeding puts pressure on the surrounding muscle fibres, reducing flexibility.

High-impact sports such as football and hockey are commonly associated with thigh contusions, but any direct trauma to the thigh can cause a contusion.

Cause of injury

Impact to the muscle from a blunt surface such as the ground, a helmet, foot etc.

Signs and symptoms

Pain and tenderness over the injured area. Swelling and bruising may be present. Pain on weightbearing and stretching of the muscle.

Complications if left unattended

Myositis ossificans, the formation of bony or calcified deposits in muscle tissue, can develop from unattended thigh contusions. Muscle ruptures can also occur when a contusion is left untreated and activity is continued.

Immediate treatment

Rest and ice. Anti-inflammatory medication. Then heat and massage to promote blood flow and healing.

Rehabilitation and prevention

After the pain subsides it is important to regain flexibility and strength in the injured muscle. Gentle stretching will improve flexibility and help to avoid scar tissue formation. While the muscle is healing, working the surrounding muscles as tolerable may help to speed recovery by increasing blood flow and limit scarring. Use of proper protective equipment during activities and avoiding impact to the thigh will help prevent thigh contusions.

Long-term prognosis

Proper treatment of a thigh contusion will ensure that there are no future complications. Flexibility and strength should return to normal after rehabilitation of the injured muscle.

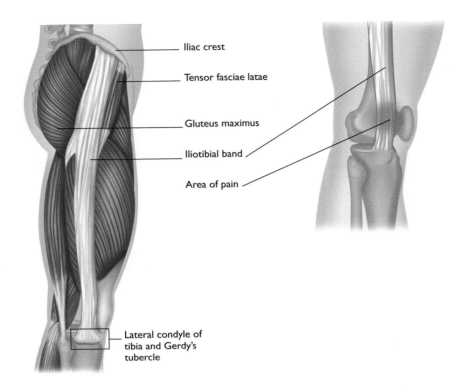

Iliac crest

Tensor fasciae latae

Gluteus maximus

Iliotibial band

Area of pain

Lateral condyle of tibia and Gerdy's tubercle

ILIOTIBIAL BAND SYNDROME

Iliotibial band (ITB) syndrome refers to excessive pulling or friction of the ITB over the greater trochanter of the femur near the hip and/or the lateral condyle at the knee. This friction or tension causes inflammation and significant pain when the knees and hips flex or extend. Bursitis can also ensue.

Cause of injury

Tension or friction of the ITB. Repetitive hip and knee flexion and extension while the tensor fasciae latae (TFL) is contracted, such as with running. Tight TFL and ITB. Muscle imbalances.

Signs and symptoms

Knee pain over the lateral condyle. Pain with flexion and extension of the knee.

Complications if left unattended

The ITB and accompanying TFL become tight due to the pain and inflammation. If left unattended this can lead to chronic pain and further injury to the knee and hip.

Immediate treatment

RICER. Anti-inflammatory medication. Then heat and massage to promote blood flow and healing.

Rehabilitation and prevention

Increasing flexibility as pain allows will help speed recovery. After the pain has subsided, increasing strength and flexibility of all the muscles of the thighs and hips to develop balance will help prevent future issues. Identifying and fixing any errors in running form will also help to prevent recurrence of the injury.

Long-term prognosis

ITB syndrome can be treated successfully with no lingering effects. Inflammation and pain may return when the activity is resumed and form corrections must be made to prevent future problems.

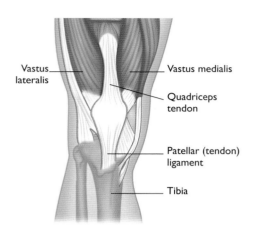

Vastus lateralis

Vastus medialis

Quadriceps tendon

Patellar (tendon) ligament

Tibia

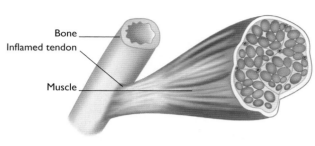

Bone

Inflamed tendon

Muscle

QUADRICEPS TENDINITIS

Inflammation of the quadriceps tendon can be a result of repetitive stress to the quadriceps or excessive stress before the muscle is conditioned. Minor tears may occur in the tendon when it is stretched while subjected to loading. Pain just above the patella (kneecap), especially when extending (straightening) the knee, usually accompanies this injury.

Cause of injury

Repetitive stress to the tendon, e.g. running or jumping. Repetitive acceleration and deceleration, e.g. hurdling or football. Untreated injury to the quadriceps.

Signs and symptoms

Pain just above the patella. Jumping, running, kneeling or walking down stairs may aggravate the pain.

Complications if left unattended

The quadriceps muscles may become stiff and shortened and the tendon will become weak if left untreated. This could lead to a rupture of the tendon. A change in gait or landing form in the case of hurdlers can lead to other injuries as well.

Immediate treatment

Rest and ice. Anti-inflammatory medication. Training modification.

Rehabilitation and prevention

Rehabilitation should include stretching and strengthening exercises for the quadriceps. Activities such as swimming can be helpful to reduce the stress on the tendon during rehabilitation. Return to a normal activity schedule should be delayed until pain subsides completely and strength is restored. Keeping the quadriceps flexible and strong will help prevent this condition.

Long-term prognosis

A full recovery with no long-term disability or lingering effects can be expected in most cases of tendinitis, and surgery is only necessary in extremely rare cases.

REHABILITATION EXERCISES

Barbell squat

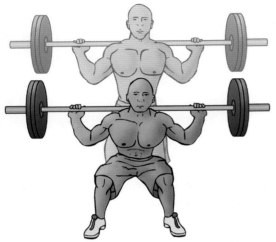

Stand with your feet shoulder width apart and a bar resting at the base of your neck. Without moving your feet, bend your knees as though you are about to sit in a chair, and slowly come back to a standing position.

Barbell lunge

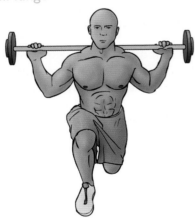

Stand with your feet shoulder width apart and a bar resting at the base of your neck. Step forward with one foot and let your opposite knee fall to the ground without letting it touch. Push yourself back up to the start position and then step forward with your other foot, letting the other knee do the same.

Barbell step-up

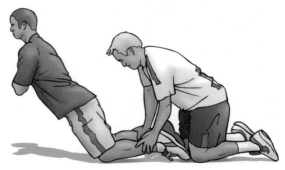

Stand in front of an elevated support or step with a barbell resting at the base of your neck. Step up onto the support with one foot and let your other foot follow. Step back down and do the same, but with your opposite foot.

Nordic curl

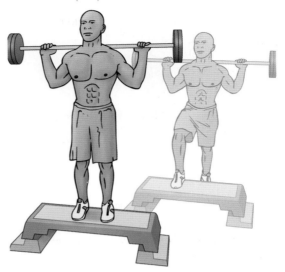

Lie on your stomach and have a friend hold your ankles. Without pressing against the floor with your hands, lift your body up to as close to a kneeling position as you can. Release and repeat.

Leg press

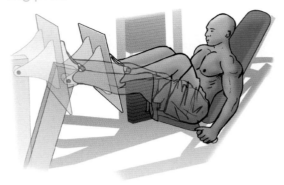

Sit on a leg press machine with your feet shoulder width apart in front of you. Press against the plate with your legs until they are nearly straight. Slowly lower to the start position and repeat.

Lying hamstring curl

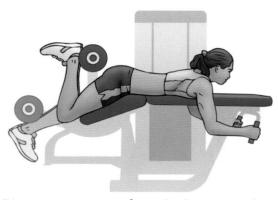

Lie on your stomach and place your feet underneath the cylinder-shaped pad. Bend your knees and lift the pad as close to your backside as possible. Slowly lower to the start position and repeat.

Lying hamstring stretch

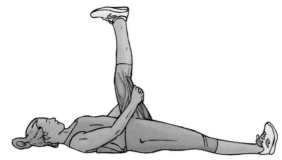

Lie on your back and bend one leg. Raise your straight leg and pull it toward your chest.

Kneeling quad stretch

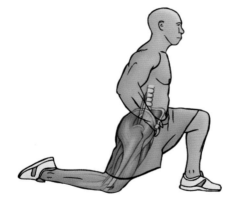

Kneel on one foot and the opposite knee. If needed, hold on to something to keep your balance. Push your hips forward.

Sports Injuries of the Knee

ANATOMY AND PHYSIOLOGY

The knee joint connects the bones of the upper and lower leg. The knee can be considered as two articulations: the patellofemoral and tibiofemoral joints. In the tibiofemoral joint the medial and lateral condyles of the femur form the top of the joint, articulating with the head of the tibia below. The patella, or kneecap, is a sesamoid bone that rests over the anterior surface of the knee joint in the groove between the femoral condyles. Just below and lateral to the knee, the head of the fibula articulates with the tibia to form the superior tibiofibular joint.

> **Note**
> *There is often confusion about whether to refer to the patellar tendon or the patellar ligament. The patellar ligament (ligamentum patellae) extends from the patella down to the tibial tuberosity. If one thinks of the patella as a bone in its own right, then it should naturally be called the patellar ligament, since it connects two bones (the patella to the tibia). However, if you consider the patella to be a sesamoid bone living within the quadriceps tendon, then calling it the patellar tendon also seems correct as it connects muscle to bone. Another suggestion might be that as a tendon ages it becomes more ligamentous. For clarity, it is referred to as the patellar (tendon) ligament throughout.*

The knee is stabilized by tough, fibrous bands of ligaments. The collateral ligaments prevent excessive side-to-side motion of the knee. The lateral collateral ligament (LCL) on the outside of the knee connects the femur to the head of the fibula. The medial collateral ligament (MCL) on the inside of the knee connects the femur to the tibia.

The posterior cruciate ligament (PCL) is located in the rear of the knee inside the fibrous joint capsule and connects the femur and the tibia. It controls backward displacement of the tibia. The anterior cruciate ligament (ACL) also lies inside the joint capsule and connects the tibia and femur in the centre of the knee. It controls rotation and forward displacement of the tibia. The LCL, MCL, PCL and ACL are the four major ligaments of the knee.

Other ligaments help add stability to the joint. The transverse ligament runs in front of the lateral and medial menisci (see below) and connects the two. The oblique and arcuate popliteal ligaments round out the ligament structure and help stabilize the posterolateral aspect of the joint.

The knee joint also contains two specialist structures called menisci, crescent-shaped wedges of fibrocartilage attached to the flat surface of the top of the tibia. Their function is to improve the fit of the joint surfaces; reduce friction between the tibia and the femur; disperse the body weight and act as shock absorbers. The menisci keep the knee joint moving smoothly and within the proper plane. They are prone to wear and tear and are often damaged in sports injuries.

The fibrous capsule of the knee joint is strengthened by the tendons of the muscles that cross the joint. The quadriceps tendon runs from the quadriceps muscles to the patella. It continues over and around the patella and becomes the patellar tendon below the bone to its attachment on the tibia. Posteriorly, the tendons of the hamstring complex run over the knee joint and connect to the tibia. The gastrocnemius tendons run up from the gastrocnemius muscle, in the posterior calf, to attach on the femoral condyles. Medially the capsule is strengthened by the combined pes anserine (duck's foot) tendon attachments of sartorius, gracilis and semitendinosus.

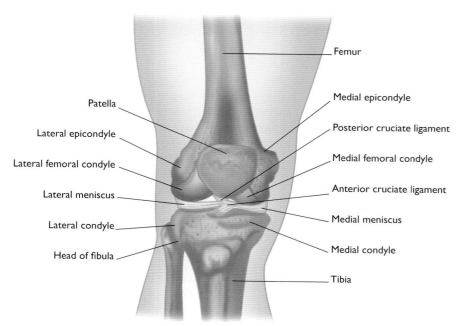

The knee joint, anterior view.

- Femur
- Medial epicondyle
- Posterior cruciate ligament
- Medial femoral condyle
- Anterior cruciate ligament
- Medial meniscus
- Medial condyle
- Tibia

- Patella
- Lateral epicondyle
- Lateral femoral condyle
- Lateral meniscus
- Lateral condyle
- Head of fibula

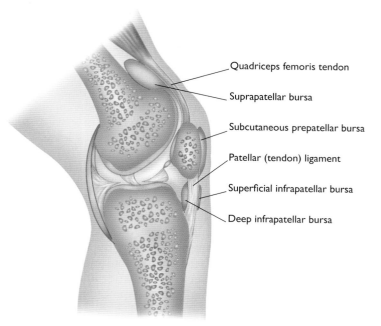

- Quadriceps femoris tendon
- Suprapatellar bursa
- Subcutaneous prepatellar bursa
- Patellar (tendon) ligament
- Superficial infrapatellar bursa
- Deep infrapatellar bursa

The knee joint, mid-sagittal view.

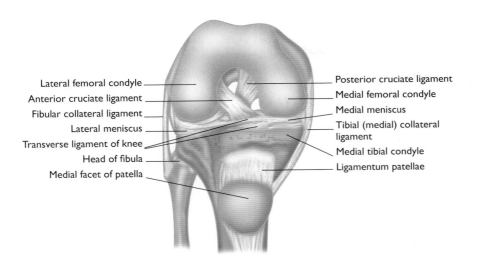

Lateral femoral condyle — Posterior cruciate ligament
Anterior cruciate ligament — Medial femoral condyle
Fibular collateral ligament — Medial meniscus
Lateral meniscus — Tibial (medial) collateral ligament
Transverse ligament of knee — Medial tibial condyle
Head of fibula — Ligamentum patellae
Medial facet of patella

The knee joint, right leg, anterior view.

The synovium is the membrane that lines the knee joint and secretes fluid for lubrication. The entire articular capsule is lined with synovium. It is responsible for keeping the joint lubricated and protecting the cartilage.

Bursae are small sacs filled with synovial fluid. They cushion and protect the bones, tendons and ligaments of the knee. There are numerous bursae around the knee, some of which are directly connected to the synovial membrane of the joint. The clinically important ones are the suprapatellar, and infrapatellar bursae anteriorly; the popliteal bursa posteriorly and the pes anserine bursa medially.

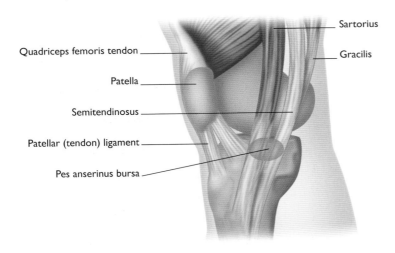

Quadriceps femoris tendon — Sartorius
Patella — Gracilis
Semitendinosus
Patellar (tendon) ligament
Pes anserinus bursa

The knee joint, medial view.

The muscles around the knee joint are responsible for movement of the upper and lower leg and stability of the knee joint. The major muscles at the front of the upper leg (or thigh) are sartorius and quadriceps, which include rectus femoris, vastus medialis, vastus intermedius and vastus lateralis. The major muscles at the back of the upper leg are the hamstrings, which include biceps femoris, semitendinosus and semimembranosus.

The major muscles on the inside of the thigh are pectineus, gracilis and the adductors, which include adductor brevis, adductor longus and adductor magnus. On the outside of the thigh are tensor fasciae latae (TFL) and, to a lesser degree, the gluteal muscles, which include gluteus maximus, gluteus medius and gluteus minimus. The major muscles of the lower leg include tibialis anterior at the front and gastrocnemius and soleus at the back.

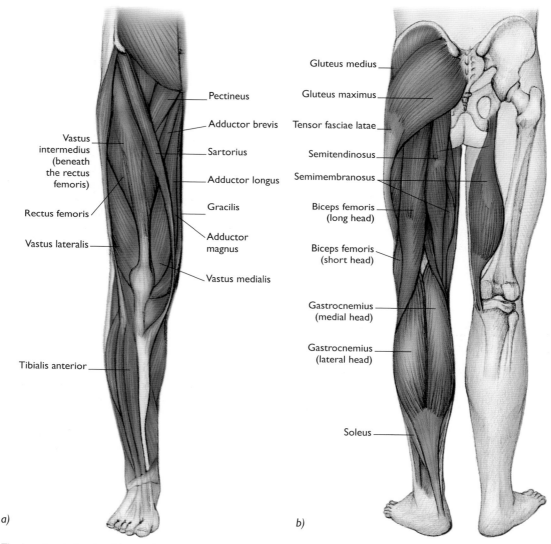

The leg; a) anterior view, b) posterior view.

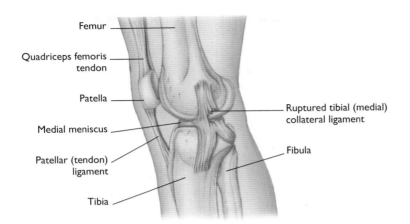

Femur

Quadriceps femoris tendon

Patella

Medial meniscus

Patellar (tendon) ligament

Tibia

Ruptured tibial (medial) collateral ligament

Fibula

MEDIAL COLLATERAL LIGAMENT SPRAIN

Medial collateral ligament sprains are usually caused by force applied to the outside of the knee joint as in a tackle in football. Force applied to the outside of the knee causes the inside of the knee to open, stretching the medial collateral ligament. The extent of the stretch determines whether the ligament simply stretches, tears partially or completely tears.

Cause of injury
Force applied to the outside of the knee joint.

Signs and symptoms
Pain over the medial portion of the knee. Swelling and tenderness. Instability in the knee and pain on weightbearing.

Complications if left unattended
The ligament, in rare cases, may repair itself but if left unattended could lead to a more severe sprain. The pain and instability in the knee may not resolve. Continued activity on the injured knee could lead to injuries in the other ligaments due to the instability.

Immediate treatment
RICER. Immobilization. Anti-inflammatory medication.

Rehabilitation and prevention
Depending on the severity of the sprain, simple rest and gradual introduction back into activity may be enough. For more severe sprains, braces may be needed during the strengthening phase of rehabilitation and the early portion of the return to activity. The most severe sprains may require extended immobilization and rest from the activity. As range of motion and strength begin to return, stationary bikes and other equipment may be used. Ensuring adequate strength in the thigh muscles and conditioning before starting any activity that is susceptible to trauma to the knee will help prevent these types of injuries.

Long-term prognosis
The ligament will usually heal with no limitations, although in some cases there is residual looseness in the medial part of the knee. Very rarely, surgery is required to repair the ligaments. Meniscal tearing may also result in a severe sprain that may require surgical repair.

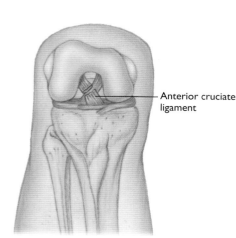

Anterior cruciate ligament

ANTERIOR COLLATERAL LIGAMENT SPRAIN

The anterior cruciate ligament (ACL) is commonly injured in sports where there are a lot of direction changes and possible impacts. Football, lacrosse and other fast-moving games often result in ACL sprains.

The most common mechanism for this injury is when the knee rotates while the foot is planted. The stress can cause a tear in the ACL which can range from minor tearing of a few fibres to a complete rupture. It can also be torn as the result of a hard blow to the knee; usually other ligaments and the meniscus are involved. Sharp pain at the time of the injury accompanied by swelling in the knee joint may be a sign of an ACL tear.

Cause of injury

Forceful twisting of the knee when the foot is planted. Occasionally a forceful blow to the knee, especially if the foot is fixed as well.

Signs and symptoms

Pain immediately that may go away. Swelling in the knee joint. Instability in the knee, especially with the tibia.

Complications if left unattended

If left unattended this injury may not heal properly. Instability in the joint could lead to injury to other ligaments. Chronic pain and instability could lead to future limitations.

Immediate treatment

RICER. Immobilization. Immediate referral to a sports medicine professional.

Rehabilitation and prevention

Once stability and strength return and pain subsides, gradual introduction of activities such as stationary biking can be undertaken. Range of motion and strengthening exercises are an important part of rehabilitation. Swimming and other non-weightbearing exercise may be used until the strength returns to normal. Strengthening the muscles of the quadriceps, hamstrings and calves will help to protect the ACL. Proper conditioning before beginning high-impact activities will also provide protection.

Long-term prognosis

ACL sprains that involve a complete tear often require surgery to reattach the ligament. Minor sprains can often be healed completely without surgery. Return to full activity may be a prolonged process and some activities may be limited.

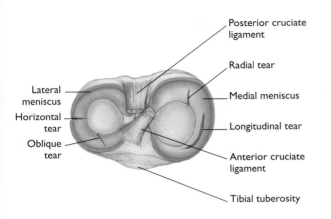

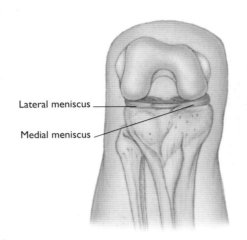

MENISCUS TEAR

Tearing of the menisci can occur with forceful twisting of the knee or may accompany other injuries such as ligament sprains. An 'unhappy triad' is when a blow to the lateral side of the knee causes tearing of the medial collateral ligament, the anterior cruciate ligament and the menisci. This is often seen in sports that require a planting of the foot to quickly change direction. The medial meniscus is injured much more frequently than the lateral meniscus, mainly due to it being more securely attached to the tibia and, therefore, less mobile.

Cause of injury
Forceful twisting of the knee joint, most commonly seen when the knee is also bent. May accompany ligament strains as well.

Signs and symptoms
Pain in the knee joint. Swelling. Catching or locking in the joint.

Complications if left unattended
A meniscal tear can cause premature wear on the cartilage at the ends of the bones and under the patella. This can lead to arthritic conditions and a fluid build-up in the knee joint. Loose pieces of cartilage and jagged edges of a damaged meniscus and can cause catching and locking.

Immediate treatment
RICER. Anti-inflammatory medication.

Rehabilitation and prevention
When recovering from a meniscal tear it is important to strengthen the muscles surrounding the knee to prevent the injury from happening again. Strong quadriceps and hamstrings help support the knee and prevent the twisting that might cause a tear. The muscles should be stretched regularly as well since tight muscles can also cause problems in the knee. After surgical repair of a meniscus tear weightbearing should be encouraged as tolerable, but as with any restart of activity should be done gradually.

Long-term prognosis
A tear to a meniscus usually requires arthroscopic surgery to repair. The surgery requires removal of the torn edges of the meniscus but leaves the main body of the meniscus intact. Therefore, most meniscus tears heal fully with no long-term limitations.

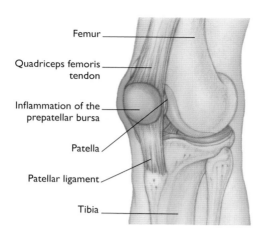

Femur

Quadriceps femoris tendon

Inflammation of the prepatellar bursa

Patella

Patellar ligament

Tibia

BURSITIS

Bursitis can be a painful condition, especially in the weightbearing knee joint. Since the job of the bursa is to cushion and lubricate the joint where friction is likely to occur, inflammation will result in pain in most weightbearing, flexion or extension activities. The knee joint has on average fourteen bursae.

The prepatellar bursa is the most commonly injured due to its superficial location. Repetitive kneeling or impact to the patella can damage this bursa. The infrapatellar bursae are most commonly inflamed during jumping and landing from repetitive friction of the patellar (tendon) ligament. The pes anserine bursa is less commonly involved in injuries but can result from load bearing on the inside of the knee, as seen with improper gait or use of worn or improperly sized running shoes. Bursae can swell as a result of fluid effusion from the knee joint itself as may be seen in the case of popliteal bursitis, also known as a Baker's cyst.

Cause of injury
Repetitive pressure or trauma to the bursa. Repetitive friction between the bursa and tendon or bone.

Signs and symptoms
Pain and tenderness. Swelling. Pain and stiffness when kneeling or walking downstairs.

Complications if left unattended
If a bursa is allowed to rupture and release its fluid the natural cushioning will be lost. The build-up of fluid will cause loss of mobility in the joint as well.

Immediate treatment
RICER. Anti-inflammatory medication.

Rehabilitation and prevention
Strengthening the muscles around the knee will help to support the joint, and increasing flexibility also will relieve some of the pressure exerted by the tendons upon the bursa. Frequent rests when required to be in a kneeling or crouching position also help to prevent this condition. Identifying any underlying problems such as improper equipment or form is important during rehabilitation to prevent bursitis from recurring.

Long-term prognosis
Bursitis is seldom a long-term concern if treated properly. Occasionally draining of the fluid from the joint is necessary.

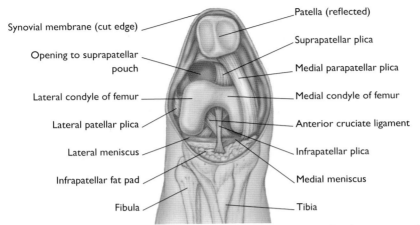

Synovial membrane (cut edge)
Opening to suprapatellar pouch
Lateral condyle of femur
Lateral patellar plica
Lateral meniscus
Infrapatellar fat pad
Fibula

Patella (reflected)
Suprapatellar plica
Medial parapatellar plica
Medial condyle of femur
Anterior cruciate ligament
Infrapatellar plica
Medial meniscus
Tibia

INFLAMMATION OF THE SYNOVIAL PLICA

The synovial plica is a thin fibrous membrane that is a remnant from the foetal knee development. The plica once divided the knee into three separate compartments during foetal development but then became a part of the knee structure as the compartments became one protective cavity.

Plica seldom cause problems by themselves but may become inflamed due to friction or pinching between the patella and the femur, common when the knee is flexed and placed under stress. This in turn causes more friction creating a vicious cycle.

Cause of injury
Trauma to the flexed knee. Repetitive stress, especially with medial weightbearing, e.g. cycling.

Signs and symptoms
Pain. Tenderness over the synovial plica.

Complications if left unattended
The synovial plica will continue to become inflamed and limit flexion activity in the knee if left unattended. The pain may also cause a change in gait or running form that could lead to other overuse injuries.

Immediate treatment
Reducing activity. RICER. Anti-inflammatory medication.

Rehabilitation and prevention
Strengthening the quadriceps and hamstrings will take pressure off the synovial plica. Increasing flexibility in these muscles will also relieve pressure that may be irritating the condition. Use of proper equipment, especially running shoes, can eliminate the irritation and force the knee back into proper alignment during activity.

Long-term prognosis
Once pain subsides, a return to normal activity can be expected. Very rarely is arthroscopic surgery required to remove the plica. No adverse effects have been found from the removal of the synovial plica and a complete return to activity can be expected.

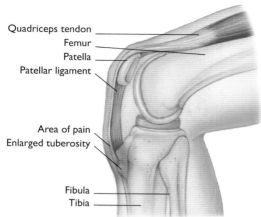

Quadriceps tendon
Femur
Patella
Patellar ligament

Area of pain
Enlarged tuberosity

Fibula
Tibia

OSGOOD-SCHLATTER DISEASE

Osgood-Schlatter disease is a traction-type injury of the tibial apophysis where the patellar (tendon) ligament pulls on the tibial tuberosity just below the knee. It is a condition that affects active young teens. It is more prevalent in males (particularly boys aged 10–15) than females and has a slightly higher prevalence in the left knee than the right. When the quadriceps is tight or there is repetitive flexion and extension this stress may cause inflammation and pain. A similar condition, Larsen-Johansson syndrome, results in pain and tenderness over the inferior pole (extremity) of the patella but is treated in a similar way to Osgood-Schlatter disease.

The bones of a developing skeleton are not as hard as mature bones. So the force of the ligament pulling up on the tibia may cause small avulsion fractures leading to inflammation and pain. The body may try to repair and protect this area by building more bone, resulting in a bony prominence just under the knee which gives the characteristic tibial bump. This is exacerbated in adolescents by a growth spurt, since the lengthening of bones often exceeds the growth of the muscles attached causing tight muscles. This puts additional force on the attached tendons. During running, jumping and kicking activities, the quadriceps must contract and relax continuously which also stresses the attachment at the tibia.

Cause of injury
Tight quadriceps due to growth spurt. Prior knee injury. Repetitive contractions of the quadriceps muscles.

Signs and symptoms
Pain, worse at full extension and during squatting, subsides with rest. Swelling over the tibial tuberosity just below the knee. Redness and inflammation of the skin just below the knee.

Complications if left unattended
If left unattended the condition will continue to cause pain and inflammation and could lead to muscle loss in the quadriceps. In rare cases, untreated Osgood-Schlatter disease could lead to a complete avulsion fracture of the tibia.

Immediate treatment
RICER. Anti-inflammatory medication.

Rehabilitation and prevention
Most cases of Osgood-Schlatter disease respond well to rest and then a regimen of stretching and strengthening the quadriceps muscles. Limiting activities that cause pain and tend to aggravate the issue is important during recovery. Gradual increases in intensity and proper warm-up techniques will help prevent this condition.

Long-term prognosis
This condition tends to correct itself as the bone becomes stronger and mature. The pain and inflammation subside and there are seldom any long-term effects. Rare cases may require corticosteroid injections to aid recovery.

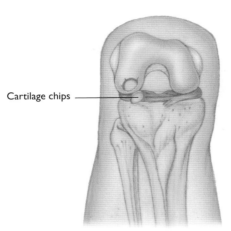

Cartilage chips

OSTEOCHONDRITIS DISSECANS

Osteochondritis dissecans occurs when a fragment of bone adjacent to the articular surface of a joint is deprived of its blood supply, leading to avascular necrosis. This causes the cartilage to become brittle and pieces, or loose bodies, may break off. Loose cartilage in the joint can cause pain and inflammation. A feeling of instability and a "clicking" or locking in the joint may be noticed. Although found in several joints, this condition is most commonly associated with the knee and is particularly prevalent in males aged 10–20 years.

Cause of injury
Loss of blood supply to the end of the bone and attached cartilage. Impact to the joint causing a tearing or breaking of the cartilage at the bone end. Repetitive friction leading to the cartilage becoming brittle and breaking away.

Signs and symptoms
Aching, diffuse pain and swelling, especially during activity. Stiffness with rest. Clicking or weakness in the joint. Momentary locking if the bony fragment has displaced and is free floating within the joint.

Complications if left unattended
If left unattended, loose bodies will continue to cause damage to the inner surface of the joint and could eventually lead to degenerative osteoarthritis. The loose bodies could also lead to tearing or "grooving" of other cartilage in the joint.

Immediate treatment
Rest and referral to a sports medicine professional. Immobilization. Anti-inflammatory medication. Positive diagnosis made with a radiograph.

Rehabilitation and prevention
Strengthening the muscles surrounding the knee will help support it better during activity. Limiting the amount of time spent doing repetitive movements may also be required. Treatment of minor injuries to the joint may also help stop the chance of the blood supply being cut off. Limit activities that cause pain and gradually work back into a full schedule.

Long-term prognosis
If the broken cartilage does not release from the bone it may repair itself. However, if it becomes lodged in the joint and the body does not dissolve it surgery may be required. In younger athletes a complete recovery and return to activity may be expected. In older athletes the development of degenerative osteoarthritis is usually a by-product of this condition.

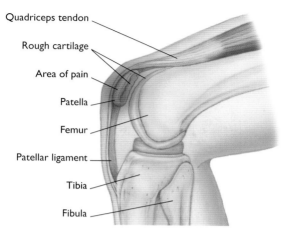

Quadriceps tendon
Rough cartilage
Area of pain
Patella
Femur
Patellar ligament
Tibia
Fibula

PATELLOFEMORAL PAIN SYNDROME

Pain in the patella (kneecap), especially after sitting for a long time or running downhill, may result from incorrect movement of the patella over the femur or tight tendons. The articular cartilage under the patella may become inflamed as well, leading to another condition called chondromalacia patellae which is found more commonly in women.

The angle formed between the two lines of pull of the quadriceps muscle and the patellar (tendon) ligament is known as the Q-angle. If the patella moves out of its normal path, even slightly, it can cause irritation and pain. Tight tendons also place pressure on the patella causing inflammation.

Cause of injury
Incorrect running form or improper shoes. Weak or tight quadriceps. Chronic patella dislocations.

Signs and symptoms
Pain on and under the patella which worsens after sitting for extended periods or walking down stairs. Clicking or grinding may be felt when flexing the knee. Dull, aching pain in the centre of the knee.

Complications if left unattended
The inflammation from this condition if left unattended can worsen and cause more permanent damage to the surrounding structures. If the tendon becomes inflamed it could eventually rupture. The cartilage under the patella may also become inflamed.

Immediate treatment
Rest and reducing exercise intensity and duration. Ice and anti-inflammatory medication.

Rehabilitation and prevention
Rehabilitation starts with restoring the strength and flexibility of the quadriceps. When returning to activity after pain has subsided, gradual increases in intensity, limiting repetitive stresses on the knee and proper warm-up techniques will ensure that the pain does not return.

Strong, flexible quadriceps and hamstrings and avoiding overuse will help prevent patellofemoral pain syndrome. A good warm-up before training will also help.

Long-term prognosis
With complete treatment there are seldom any long-lasting effects. If the condition does not respond to treatment surgical intervention may be necessary.

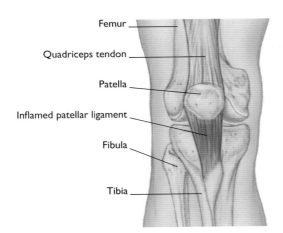

Femur
Quadriceps tendon
Patella
Inflamed patellar ligament
Fibula
Tibia

PATELLAR TENDINITIS

Activities that require repetitive jumping like basketball or volleyball can lead to tendinitis in the patellar (tendon) ligament, also referred to as jumper's knee. The force placed on the tendon over time can lead to inflammation and pain. The pain is generally felt just below the patella (kneecap).

Patellar tendinitis affects the teno-osseous junction of the quadriceps tendon as it attaches to the superior pole of the patella and the patellar (tendon) ligament as it attaches to the inferior pole of the patella and the tibial tuberosity. Pain is concentrated on the patellar (tendon) ligament but can also occur at the insertion of the patellar (tendon) ligament into the tibial tuberosity. The patellar (tendon) ligament is involved in straightening the knee. It is also the first area to experience shock when landing from a jump. It is forced to stretch as the quadriceps contracts to slow down the flexion of the knee. This repetitive stress can lead to minor trauma to the tendon which will lead to inflammation. Repetitive flexion and extension of the knee also place stress on this tendon if the tendon does not travel in the required path.

Cause of injury
Repetitive jumping and landing activities. Running and kicking activities. Untreated minor injury to the patellar tendon.

Signs and symptoms
Pain and inflammation of the patellar tendon, especially from repetitive or eccentric knee extension activity or kneeling. Swelling and tenderness around the tendon.

Complications if left unattended
As with most tendinitis, inflammation that is left untreated will cause additional irritation, setting up a vicious cycle. This can eventually lead to a rupture of the tendon. Damage to surrounding tissue may also occur.

Immediate treatment
RICER. Anti-inflammatory medication.

Rehabilitation and prevention
Stretching the quadriceps, hamstrings and calves will help relieve pressure on the patellar tendon. During rehabilitation it is important to identify the conditions that caused the injury in the first place. Thorough warm-up and proper conditioning can help prevent the onset of this condition. A support strap placed below the knee may be needed at first to support the tendon during the initial return to activity. Prevention of this condition requires strong quadriceps and a good balance of strength between the muscles that surround the knee.

Long-term prognosis
Complete recovery without lingering effects can be expected with rehabilitation and treatment. Occasionally it may return due to a weakened tendon, especially in older athletes.

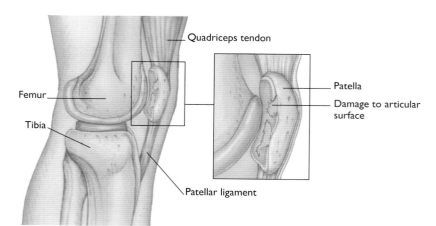

Quadriceps tendon

Femur

Tibia

Patella

Damage to articular surface

Patellar ligament

CHONDROMALACIA PATELLAE

Softening and degeneration of the articular cartilage of the patella in athletes is usually a result of overuse, trauma or abnormal forces on the knee. In older adults it can be a result of arthritis. Pain under the patella and a grating sensation when the knee is straightened are signs of this condition.

The underside of the patella is protected by thick articular (hyaline) cartilage, which is made up of collagen fibres and water. The cartilage can become damaged and softened by repetitive micro-trauma due to overuse or abnormal load bearing on the knee. This degeneration makes the surface rough which causes additional inflammation and pain. It is described in four progressive stages, from softening and blistering, to full cartilage defects and exposure of the subchondral bone.

Cause of injury
Repetitive micro-trauma to the cartilage through overuse. Misalignment of the patella. Previous fracture or dislocation of the patella.

Signs and symptoms
Pain that worsens after sitting for prolonged periods or when using stairs or rising from a seated position. Tenderness over the patella. Grating or grinding sensation when the knee is extended.

Complications if left unattended
Cartilage that degenerates and becomes rough can cause scarring on the bone surface it rubs against. This in turn causes more inflammation. Cartilage can also be torn when it is rough leading to loose bodies in the joint.

Immediate treatment
Rest and ice. Anti-inflammatory medication.

Rehabilitation and prevention
Limiting activity until the pain subsides and gradual return to exercise is advised. Strengthening and stretching the quadriceps is important to relieve pressure on the patella. Activities that increase the pain, such as deep knee bending, should be avoided until completely pain free. Avoid abnormal stress on the knee and keep the hamstrings and quadriceps strong and flexible to prevent this condition.

Long-term prognosis
Chondromalacia patellae commonly responds well to therapy and anti-inflammatory medication. In rare cases surgery may be required to correct a misalignment of the patella.

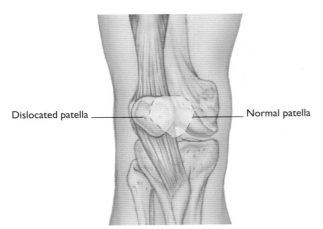

Dislocated patella —————— —————— Normal patella

PATELLAR DISLOCATION

A subluxation or dislocation of the patella (kneecap) commonly occurs during deceleration, for example when slowing from a run to a walk. The patella slides partially out of the groove between the femoral condyles but does not limit mobility. Pain and swelling may accompany this condition. Athletes who have a muscle imbalance or a structural deformity, such as a high patella, have a higher chance of subluxation.

If the outer muscle of the quadriceps, vastus lateralis, is stronger than the inner muscle, vastus medialis, the imbalance may cause an uneven tension on the patella, pulling it out of alignment. In addition, the lateral femoral condyle and patella may be bruised. This happens with forceful contractions such as planting, changing direction or landing from a jump.

Cause of injury
Strength imbalance between the outer and inner quadriceps. Impact to the side of the patella. Twisting of the knee.

Signs and symptoms
Feeling of pressure under the patella. Pain and swelling behind the patella. Pain when bending or straightening the knee.

Complications if left unattended
Continued subluxations can cause small fractures in the patella, cartilage tears and put stress on the tendons. Failure to treat a subluxation could lead to chronic subluxations.

Immediate treatment
RICER. Anti-inflammatory medication.

Rehabilitation and prevention
During rehabilitation activities that do not aggravate the injury should be sought, such as swimming or biking instead of running. Strengthening of vastus medialis and stretching vastus lateralis will help correct the muscle imbalance that may cause this condition. A brace to hold the patella in place may be needed when initially returning to activity. To prevent subluxations it is important to keep the muscles surrounding the knee strong and flexible and avoid direct impact to the patella.

Long-term prognosis
Subluxations respond well to rest, rehabilitation and anti-inflammatory measures. Rarely surgery may be required to prevent recurring subluxations due to misalignment or instability.

REHABILITATION EXERCISES

Leg extension

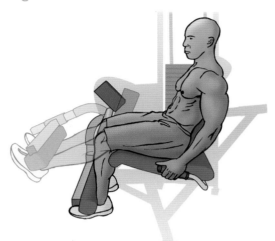

Sit down and put the tops of your feet behind the cylinder-shaped pad. Push against it until your legs are nearly straight. Slowly lower to the start position and Repeat.

Dumbbell walking lunge

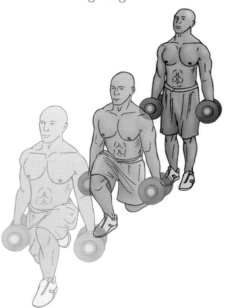

With a dumbbell in each hand, lunge forward with one foot letting your opposite knee almost touch the ground. Instead of returning to your original position, step forward with your back leg and lunge letting your other knee almost touch the ground. Continue.

Dumbbell step up

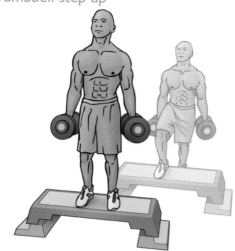

With a dumbbell in each hand, step up onto an elevated support or step. Step down and step back up with your other foot.

Wall sit

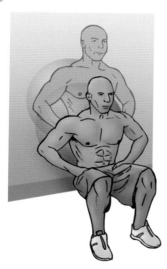

Stand straight up with a gym ball placed between your back and on a wall. Slide downward with the gym ball rolling down the wall until you are in a sitting position. Hold the position for a second and then raise up into the standing position.

Stationary bike

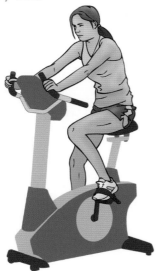

Sit comfortably on a stationary bike with your hands gripping the handlebars. Place your feet securely on the pedals and rotate them.

Lateral side stretch

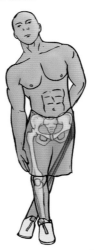

Stand upright and cross one foot behind the other. Lean toward the foot that is behind the other.

Standing quad stretch

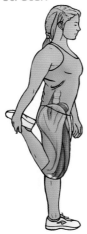

Stand upright while balancing on one leg. Pull your other foot up behind your buttocks and keep your knees together while pushing your hips forward. Hold on to something for balance.

15 Sports Injuries of the Shin and Calf

ANATOMY AND PHYSIOLOGY

The tibia (shin bone) is the larger and more medial of the bones of the lower leg. At its proximal end, the medial and lateral condyles articulate with the distal end of the femur to form the knee joint. The tibial tuberosity is a roughened area on the anterior surface of the tibia and the medial malleolus can be felt as the inner bone (medial malleolus) of the ankle. The tibia is the weightbearing bone of the lower leg and therefore takes a large amount of the force of impact during running and jumping activities.

The fibula lies lateral and parallel to the tibia and is thin and stick-like. The fibula is not a weightbearing bone but is an important point for muscle attachment. The distal head of the fibula can be felt as the lateral malleolus of the ankle.

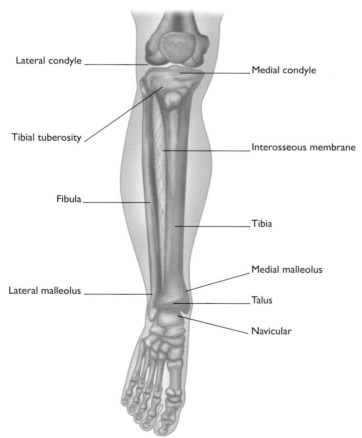

Tibia and fibula of the right leg, anterior view.

Muscles of the posterior calf include gastrocnemius and soleus, known as the triceps surae, and plantaris. These muscles attach to the foot via the Achilles tendon. These muscles are responsible for plantarflexing the foot at the ankle joint, enabling jumping, pushing off from a planted foot and rising up on tiptoes. The tibialis anterior muscle originates from the lateral condyle of the tibia and inserts into the medial and plantar surfaces of the bones of the medial arch. Tibialis anterior is responsible for dorsiflexing the foot and is used during running and walking to 'toe up' with each step. Together with tibialis posterior, tibialis anterior inverts the foot and ankle while laterally the peroneal muscles are responsible for eversion.

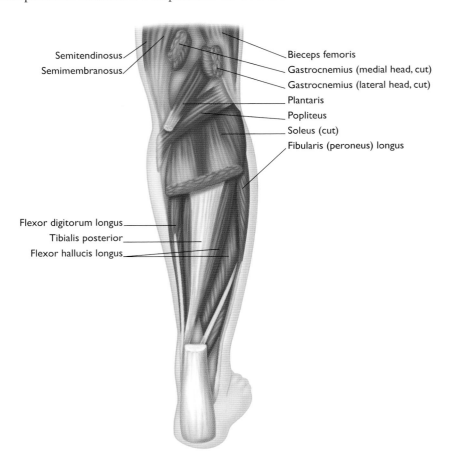

The calf muscles, right leg, posterior view.

The Achilles tendon is the largest tendon in the body, being approximately 15 centimetres long and 2 centimetres thick. Taking its name from the mythical Greek warrior Achilles, it originates from the musculo-tendinous junction of the calf muscles and inserts into the posterior aspect of the calcaneus (heel bone). The tendon is separated from the calcaneus by the retrocalcaneal bursa and from the skin by the subcutaneous calcaneal bursa. It plantarflexes the foot at the ankle when the calf muscles contract. The Achilles tendon is well known for its vulnerability to sports injury.

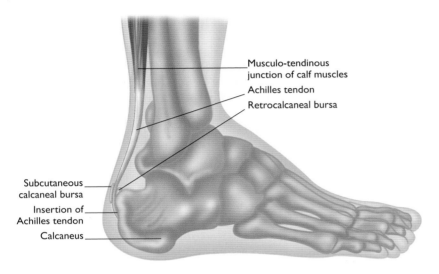

The Achilles tendon.

FRACTURES (TIBIA, FIBULA)

The tibia and fibula have outer shells of cortical bone with cancellous bone underneath. Cortical bone is stiffer and capable of withstanding great stress. When the outer shell is cracked it is called a fracture. The bone may be either partially fractured or completely broken.

Although either the tibia or fibula can be fractured alone they are most commonly fractured together. Most fractures involve the proximal (near the knee) or distal (near the ankle) ends of the bone. Due to the thin covering of skin and other tissue over the tibia these fractures are often open fractures meaning the broken bone ends break the skin.

Cause of injury

Direct force (impact) to the bones along the shaft or extreme loading of the bone, such as landing from a high fall. Rotational or indirect forces on the bones, e.g. tackle in football. Twisting, especially when the bone is under load or when the foot is fixed.

Signs and symptoms

Pain, inability to walk or bear weight and often inability to move the leg. Deformity may be present at the fracture site or the fracture may be open (see above). Swelling and tenderness.

Complications if left unattended

Instability in the lower leg is one long-term complication of an untreated fracture. Blood vessel damage from a fracture can lead to internal bleeding and swelling as well as circulation problems for the foot. Nerve involvement can lead to serious problems such as drop foot or loss of sensation in the lower leg and foot.

Immediate treatment

Immobilize the leg. Control any bleeding that might be present with an open fracture. Seek medical attention immediately.

Rehabilitation and prevention

After the fracture has healed it will be necessary to rebuild the strength and flexibility of the muscles of the lower leg. Range of motion activities may be needed for the knee and ankle depending on the location of the fracture and the extent of immobilization required. When the fracture has healed a gradual re-entry into activity must be observed to prevent re-injury. Strong calf and tibialis anterior muscles will help protect the tibia and fibula.

Long-term prognosis

If set properly and allowed to heal fully, a fracture should not present any future problems. In some cases a rod or pins may be needed to hold the bones in place during healing. Surgery may be required in a few cases where blood vessel or nerve damage is severe.

CALF STRAIN

Failure to warm-up properly can lead to calf strains. The calf muscles are used when taking off during a sprint, jumping, changing directions or standing up from a deep squat. These are usually explosive movements requiring forceful contractions of the calf muscles. Strains can result from incorrect foot positioning during activity or an eccentric contraction beyond the strength level of the muscle.

When taking off and changing direction the calf muscles are particularly vulnerable to tearing at their junction with the tendon. An eccentric contraction, a contraction while the muscle stretches such as when landing from a jump, can also cause a tear if the muscle is fatigued or not strong enough to bear the load placed on it.

Cause of injury

Forceful contraction of gastrocnemius or soleus. Forceful eccentric contraction. Improper foot position when pushing off or landing.

Signs and symptoms

Pain in the calf muscle, usually mid-calf. Pain when standing on tiptoes and sometimes pain when bending the knee. Swelling or bruising in the calf.

Complications if left unattended

Any strain left unattended can lead to a complete rupture. The calf muscles are used when standing and walking so pain can become disabling. A limp or change in gait due to this injury could lead to injury in other areas.

Immediate treatment

RICER. Anti-inflammatory medication. Then heat and massage to promote blood flow and healing.

Rehabilitation and prevention

As the pain subsides, a programme of light stretching may help facilitate healing. When the pain has subsided, strengthening and stretching will help to prevent future injury. Proper warm-up before activities will help protect the muscle from tears. Strong, flexible muscles resist strains better and recover more quickly.

Long-term prognosis

Muscle strains, when treated properly with rest and therapy, seldom have lingering effects. In very rare cases where the muscle detaches completely, surgery may be required to re-attach the muscle.

ACHILLES TENDON STRAIN

Achilles tendon strains can be very painful and require significant healing time. An injury to this tendon can be debilitating because of its involvement in walking and even balance during weightbearing. Explosive activities such as sprinting and jumping, and activities that involve pushing against resistance such as rugby and weight training, contribute greatly to this injury.

The strain can be graded on a scale from 1 to 3:

Grade 1 strain: Stretching or minor tear of less than 25% of the tendon.
Grade 2 strain: 25–75% tearing of the tendon fibres.
Grade 3 strain: 75–100% rupture of the tendon fibres.

Cause of injury
Abrupt, forceful contraction of the calf muscles, especially when the muscle and tendon are either cold or inflexible. Excessive force applied to the foot forcing the ankle upward into dorsiflexion.

Signs and symptoms
Pain in the Achilles tendon, from mild discomfort in grade 1 strains to severe, debilitating pain in grade 3 strains. Swelling and tenderness. Pain when rising on the toes. Inability to bend the ankle. Stiffness in the calf and heel area after resting.

Complications if left unattended
A minor tear may become a complete rupture if left unattended. Bursitis and tendinitis may develop from the inflamed tendon rubbing over the heel.

Immediate treatment
RICER. Anti-inflammatory medication. Then heat and massage to promote blood flow and healing. Immobilization and medical help for grade 3 strains.

Rehabilitation and prevention
Rest is important and a gradual return to activity must be undertaken. Stretching and strengthening the calf muscles is important to rehabilitation and to prevent recurrence. Warming-up the calf muscles properly before all activities, especially those involving forceful contractions such as sprinting, is essential to prevent strains.

Long-term prognosis
Due to the lower blood supply in tendons, they take longer to heal than the muscle, but with rest and rehabilitation the Achilles tendon can return to normal function. Severe ruptures usually require surgical repair.

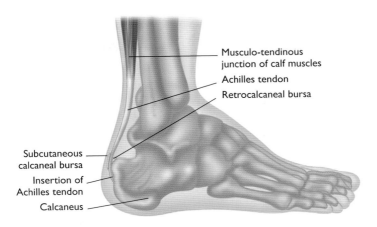

Musculo-tendinous junction of calf muscles

Achilles tendon

Retrocalcaneal bursa

Subcutaneous calcaneal bursa

Insertion of Achilles tendon

Calcaneus

ACHILLES TENDINITIS

The Achilles tendon crosses the back of the heel, which means it rides over the bone as the muscle contracts and stretches. Inflammation of the Achilles tendon can be very painful; all of the body's weight is supported by this structure and footwear often presses against this area. Repetitive stress to the tendon can lead to inflammation that causes additional irritation and further inflammation.

Activities such as basketball, running, volleyball and other running and jumping sports can lead to Achilles tendinitis. Repetitive contraction of the muscles in the calf and improper footwear or excessive pronation of the feet can lead to inflammation in the tendon.

Cause of injury
Repetitive stress from running and jumping activities. Improper footwear or awkward landing pattern of the foot during running. Untreated injuries to the calf or Achilles tendon.

Signs and symptoms
Pain and tenderness in the tendon. Swelling may be present. Contraction of the calf muscle causes pain; running and jumping may be difficult.

Complications if left unattended
Inflammation in the tendon can lead to deterioration of the tendon and eventual rupture if left untreated. Inflammation may lead to tightening of the tendon and attached muscle which could lead to tearing.

Immediate treatment
Rest, reducing or discontinuing the offending activity. Ice. Anti-inflammatory medication. Then heat and massage to promote blood flow and healing.

Rehabilitation and prevention
After a period of rest, usually lasting 5–10 days, gentle stretching and strengthening exercises can be initiated. Heat may be used on the tendon before activity to warm the tendon properly. Adequate warm-up, along with strengthening and stretching exercises for the calves, will help prevent tendinitis of the Achilles tendon.

Long-term prognosis
Tendinitis seldom has lingering effects if treated properly. Tendinitis may take from five days to several weeks to heal but rarely needs surgery to repair it.

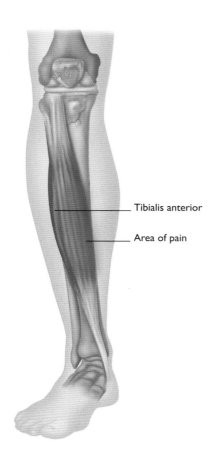

Tibialis anterior

Area of pain

MEDIAL TIBIAL PAIN SYNDROME (SHIN SPLINTS)

Shin splints are a common complaint of runners and other athletes who have just taken up running. Shin splints is a term used to cover all pain in the anterior shin area but there are several possible causes. Medial tibial pain syndrome, the most common cause of shin pain, refers to pain felt over the shin bone from irritation of the tendons that cover the shin and their attachment to the bones. Changes in duration, frequency or intensity of running can lead to this condition.

When the muscle and tendon becomes inflamed and irritated through overuse or improper form, it will cause pain in the front of the shin. Repetitive pounding on the lower leg, such as with running, can also lead to pain in the shin.

Cause of injury
Repetitive stress on the tibialis anterior muscle leading to inflammation at its bony attachment to the tibia. Repetitive impact forces on the tibia, as with running and jumping.

Signs and symptoms
Dull, aching pain over the inside of the tibia. Pain is worse with activity. Tenderness over the inner side of the tibia with possible slight swelling.

Complications if left unattended
If left unattended, shin splints can cause extreme pain and cause cessation of running activities. The inflammation can lead to other injuries including compartment syndrome.

Immediate treatment
RICER. Anti-inflammatory medication. Then heat and massage to promote blood flow and healing.

Rehabilitation and prevention
It is important to use low-impact activities, such as swimming or cycling, to maintain conditioning levels while recovering. Stretching tibialis anterior will aid recovery. To prevent this condition from developing try alternating high-impact activity days with lower-impact days. It is also important to strengthen the muscles of the lower leg to help absorb the shock of impact activities.

Long-term prognosis
Medial tibial pain syndrome can be effectively treated with no long-term effects. Only in rare cases does the condition fail to respond to rest and rehabilitation, leading to chronic inflammation and pain. Surgery may be required in those rare cases.

STRESS FRACTURE

Repetitive impact activities, such as running and jumping, can cause small cracks in the bone called stress fractures. These most often occur in the weightbearing bone, the tibia, of the lower leg.

Ground forces are transferred up the length of the tibia. Bones are constantly remodelling and rebuilding, leading to the removal of calcium from one area of the bone to build another, causing a relatively weak area. When impact is transferred up the shaft and encounters a weak area, due to either bone remodelling or a prior stress fracture, the bone may crack slightly. Over time this may lead to a more serious crack or fracture. Fatigued muscles also contribute to the possibility of stress fractures. The muscles are meant to take some of the shock away from the bones but a fatigued muscle is a poor shock absorber.

Athletes with lower bone density, due to dietary insufficiency or genetic predisposition, are more susceptible, as are athletes who train on hard surfaces at increased distance and duration. Women are more susceptible to this injury than men due to bone density deficiency conditions such as irregular or absent menstrual cycles, eating disorders or osteoporosis.

Cause of injury
Repetitive stress on the bone through impact activities such as running or jumping. Low bone density. Muscle fatigue leading to lower shock absorption by the muscles.

Signs and symptoms
Pain on weightbearing that worsens with activity and diminishes with rest. Pain is most severe at the early stage of activity, subsiding in the middle and returning at the end. Point tenderness and some swelling possible.

Complications if left unattended
If left unattended a stress fracture can become a complete fracture and lead to complications such as bleeding and nerve compromise. The pain from an untreated stress fracture may require complete cessation of activity and cause further injury to surrounding tissues.

Immediate treatment
RICER. Anti-inflammatory medication. If any instability is noted in the lower leg, or inability to bear weight, a sports medicine professional should be consulted.

Rehabilitation and prevention
During the recovery phase it is important to maintain fitness levels by using low- or non-impact activities such as swimming or biking. Strengthening the muscles of the lower leg will aid shock absorption. Warming-up properly and using cross training techniques to limit impact on the bone will help prevent stress fractures.

Long-term prognosis
Stress fractures generally heal completely with rest. Returning to activity too soon may cause a recurrence. Very rarely, surgical intervention may be needed to strengthen the bone at the fracture site.

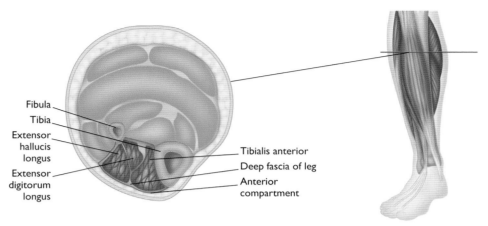

Fibula
Tibia
Extensor hallucis longus
Extensor digitorum longus

Tibialis anterior
Deep fascia of leg
Anterior compartment

ANTERIOR COMPARTMENT SYNDROME

Muscles are covered by an inflexible fibrous sleeve called fascia. Fascia creates a compartment for the muscle, with bone forming one side and the fascia covering the other sides. In the lower leg the two bones, the tibia and the fibula, create a more rigid compartment. The tibialis anterior muscle runs over the tibia and fibula and is enclosed by the fascia. Anterior compartment syndrome is usually caused by swelling or enlargement of tibialis anterior in in the anterior compartment of the lower leg. Increased intramuscular swelling, as a result of trauma or overuse, creates pressure inside the compartment which impedes blood flow and muscle function. The nerves in the compartment may be compressed causing numbness and weakness in the foot. Anterior compartment syndrome is more often a chronic rather than an acute injury. Runners and other athletes involved in activities that require a lot of repetitive flexion and extension of the foot are most susceptible.

Pain, especially when dorsiflexing the ankle to lift the foot or when raising the toes, and decreased sensation and weakness in the foot may be experienced. Virtually any injury involving bleeding or local swelling may lead to compartment syndrome.

Cause of injury
Acute: trauma to the tibialis anterior muscle causing bleeding and/or swelling.
Chronic: overuse of the muscle causing inflammation and swelling and increased pressure in the compartment. Rapid growth of the muscle before its fascial envelope can expand (as seen with anabolic steroid use).

Signs and symptoms
Pain and tightness in the shin (especially the lateral side). Worsens with exercise. Decreased sensation on top of the foot over the second toe. Weakness and tingling in the foot.

Complications if left unattended
Raised pressure in the compartment may lead to permanent nerve and blood vessel damage if left unattended. The underlying cause of the condition will most likely continue to cause irritation and swelling if not treated.

Immediate treatment
Rest, ice and elevation (no compression). Anti-inflammatory medication. Sports massage may be used to stretch the fascia.

Rehabilitation and prevention
Stretching the muscles in the front of the shin will help to alleviate some of the pressure and elongate the muscle. Massage to stretch the fascia may also help to speed recovery. Gradual strengthening and a good flexibility program will help prevent this condition. Avoiding direct trauma to the shin area will prevent acute compartment syndrome.

Long-term prognosis
If treated before damage to the nerves and blood vessels becomes serious, the recovery rate is very good. Acute or severe chronic anterior compartment syndrome may require surgical intervention to relieve the pressure in the compartment.

REHABILITATION EXERCISES

Standing calf raise

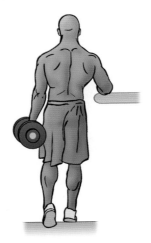

With a dumbbell in one hand and your opposite hand holding on to a support, place your toes on the edge of a step and let your heel lower toward the ground. Slowly raise up by straightening your ankle. Slowly lower yourself to the start position, repeat and then switch sides.

Seated calf raise

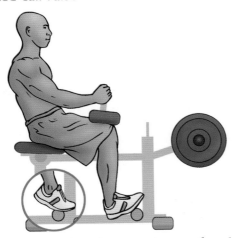

In a seated position place your toes on the edge of the step and your knees securely under the padded weight. Slowly raise the weight up by straightening your ankles, then lower the weight to the start position and repeat.

Squat jump

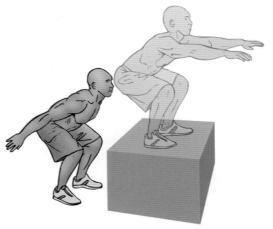

Keeping your feet shoulder width apart, bring your arms behind you and bend your knees. Jump forward bringing your knees and feet up and onto the box. Carefully step off the box and repeat.

Single legged deadlift

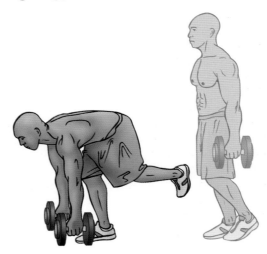

Stand upright with a dumbbell in each hand resting at your side. Balance on one leg with a slightly bent knee. Slowly lean forward at your waist moving the dumbbells toward the ground and letting your other leg move backward behind you. Raise your body back up to the start position and repeat.

Heel back calf stretch

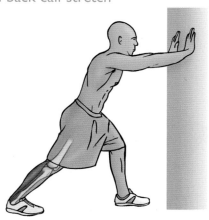

Stand upright and lean against a wall. Place one foot as far from the wall as is comfortable and make sure that both toes are facing forward and your heel is on the ground. Keep your back leg straight and lean toward the wall.

Achilles stretch

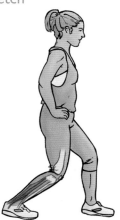

Stand upright and take one big step backward. Bend your back leg and push your heel toward the ground.

16 Sports Injuries of the Ankle

ANATOMY AND PHYSIOLOGY

The talocrural or ankle joint is a hinge joint and comprises the tibia, fibula and the talus and calcaneus bones of the foot. Its main function is to allow flexion and extension of the foot. The calcaneus or heel bone sits beneath the talus. The talus articulates proximally with the tibia and fibula at the talocrural joint and distally with the calcaneus at the subtalar joint. The dome-like articular surface of the talus is covered with cartilage to cushion and protect it. The navicular, medial cuneiform, intermediate cuneiform, lateral cuneiform and cuboid constitute the other five tarsal bones.

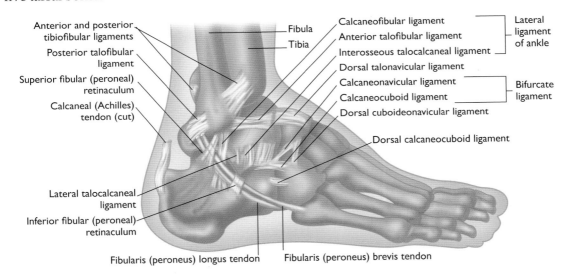

The right ankle, lateral view.

The ankle is stabilized by strong collateral ligaments. Medially the deltoid ligament protects against eversion strains. The three bands of the lateral collateral ligament run between the fibula, talus and calcaneus. Posterior and anterior ligaments connect the tibia and fibula.

The tibialis posterior tendon runs behind the medial malleolus (the inner bony prominence) of the ankle and has many points of attachment to the bones under the medial arch of the foot. This tendon supports the arch and aids in inversion of the foot. The tendons of peroneus longus and peroneus brevis run from the peroneal muscles to the foot. They pass in a groove behind the lateral malleolus (the outer bony prominence of the ankle) and attach beneath the medial arch and to the first and fifth metatarsal bones. They are held in place by a sheath that is reinforced by a band of ligament. These tendons, along with the peroneal muscles, help to stabilize the ankle and assist the calf muscles in plantarflexion.

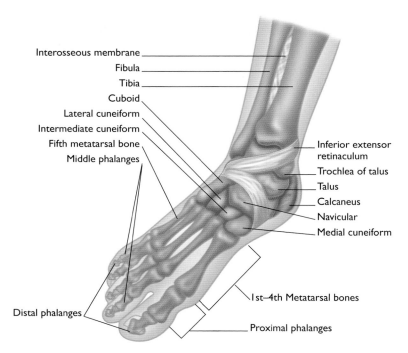

Interosseous membrane

Fibula

Tibia

Cuboid

Lateral cuneiform

Intermediate cuneiform

Fifth metatarsal bone

Middle phalanges

Inferior extensor retinaculum

Trochlea of talus

Talus

Calcaneus

Navicular

Medial cuneiform

1st–4th Metatarsal bones

Distal phalanges

Proximal phalanges

The bones of the right foot, anteromedial view.

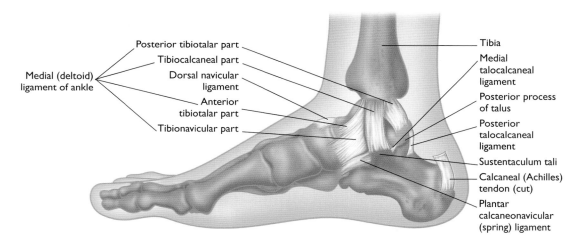

Posterior tibiotalar part

Tibiocalcaneal part

Dorsal navicular ligament

Medial (deltoid) ligament of ankle

Anterior tibiotalar part

Tibionavicular part

Tibia

Medial talocalcaneal ligament

Posterior process of talus

Posterior talocalcaneal ligament

Sustentaculum tali

Calcaneal (Achilles) tendon (cut)

Plantar calcaneonavicular (spring) ligament

The right ankle, medial view.

Flexor digitorum longus (FDL), flexor hallucis longus (FHL) and tibialis posterior lie in the deep posterior compartment of the lower leg. FDL and FHL flex the toes. Tibialis posterior is the deepest muscle and, with FHL, helps maintain the medial arch of the foot. The peroneus longus and peroneus brevis muscles lie in the lateral compartment of the lower leg. Both these muscles plantarflex and evert the foot and help prevent inversion sprains. The course of the tendon of insertion of peroneus longus helps maintain the transverse and lateral longitudinal arches of the foot.

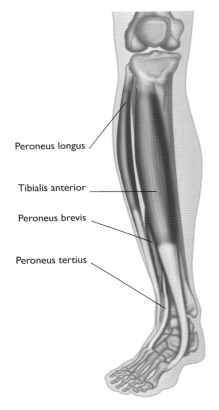
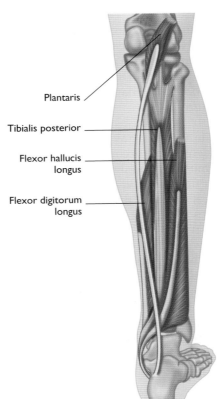

The lower calf muscles, posterior view.

ANKLE FRACTURE

Due to the ankle's involvement in all running and jumping activities it is very susceptible to injury. The majority of athletes have experienced at least a minor sprain of the ankle. Ankle fractures are less common but are nonetheless more common than other fractures. Running or jumping on uneven or changing surfaces can lead to ankle fractures. High-impact sports such as football and rugby, where the possibility of forceful twisting of the ankle may occur, also have a high incidence of ankle fractures.

In an ankle fracture, any or all of the bones and ligaments may become involved. Ankle fractures most commonly involve the ends of the tibia or fibula, or both, with some ligament stretching and tearing present as well.

Cause of injury
Forceful twisting or rolling of the ankle can cause the ends of the bones to fracture. Forceful impact to the medial or lateral side of the ankle while the foot is planted.

Signs and symptoms
Painful to touch. Swelling and discolouration. Inability to weightbear. Deformity may be present in the joint.

Complications if left unattended
An ankle fracture that is left unattended can result in incorrect or incomplete healing of the bones. Continued walking or running on the injured ankle could result in further damage to the ligaments, blood vessels and nerves that pass through the joint.

Immediate treatment
Stop the activity. Immobilize the joint and apply ice. Seek medical attention.

Rehabilitation and prevention
While the ankle is immobilized it is important to keep conditioning levels up by using upper body exercises and weight training. When cleared for activity with the ankle, strengthening and stretching of the muscles of the lower leg is essential for a speedy recovery. An ankle brace may be needed for support during the initial return to activity. Stronger calf and anterior compartment muscles help support the ankle and prevent or lessen the incidence of injuries. Avoid running and jumping on uneven surfaces as much as possible.

Long-term prognosis
Although people who have fractured their ankle tend to have a slightly higher rate of re-injury, proper strengthening and rehabilitation usually lead to a full recovery. Compound fractures or fractures resulting in bony misalignment may require surgical pinning to hold the bone in place while it heals.

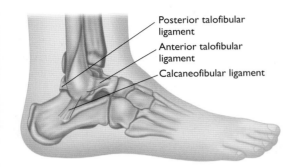

Posterior talofibular ligament
Anterior talofibular ligament
Calcaneofibular ligament

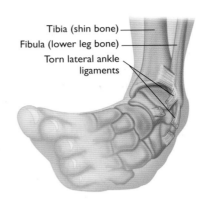

Tibia (shin bone)
Fibula (lower leg bone)
Torn lateral ankle ligaments

ANKLE SPRAIN

Anyone involved in athletics is susceptible to an ankle sprain, an acute injury to any or all of the ligaments that support the ankle structure. Tearing or stretching of the ligaments can occur when the foot is rolled or twisted forcefully. High-impact sports involving jumping, sprinting or running on changing or uneven surfaces often lead to ankle sprains. Basketball, football, cross country and hockey are a few of the sports commonly associated with ankle sprains.

Lateral ankle or inversion sprains commonly occur when stress is applied to the ankle during plantarflexion. The anterior talofibular ligament is most commonly injured. The medial malleolus may act as a fulcrum to further injure the calcaneofibular ligament if the strain continues. The peroneal tendons may absorb some of this strain. Medial ankle sprains are less common because of the strong deltoid ligament and bony structure of the ankle. When ligaments are stretched beyond their normal range some tearing of the fibres may occur.

Cause of injury
Sudden twisting of the foot. Rolling or force to the foot, most commonly laterally.

Signs and symptoms
First-degree sprains: Little or no swelling; mild pain and stiffness in the joint.
Second-degree sprains: Moderate swelling and stiffness; moderate to severe pain; difficulty weightbearing and some instability in the joint.

Third-degree sprains: Severe swelling and pain; inability to weightbear; instability and loss of function in the joint.

Complications if left unattended
Chronic pain and instability in the ankle joint may result if left unattended. Loss of strength and flexibility and possible loss of function may also result. Increased risk of re-injury.

Immediate treatment
RICER. Second- and third-degree sprains may require immobilization and immediate medical attention should be sought.

Rehabilitation and prevention
Strengthening the muscles of the lower leg is important to prevent future sprains. Balance training will help to improve proprioception (the body's awareness of movement and joint position sense) and strengthen the weakened ligaments. Flexibility exercises to reduce stiffness and improve mobility are needed also. Bracing during the initial return to activity may be needed but should not replace strengthening and flexibility development.

Long-term prognosis
With proper rehabilitation and strengthing the athlete should not experience any limitations. A slight increase in the probability of injuring that ankle may occur. Athletes who continue to experience difficulty with the ankle may need additional medical interventions including, in rare cases, possible surgery to tighten the ligaments.

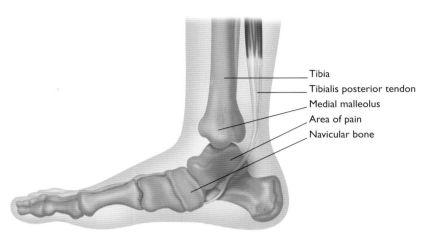

Tibia
Tibialis posterior tendon
Medial malleolus
Area of pain
Navicular bone

TIBIALIS POSTERIOR TENDINITIS

Pain along the medial (inner) side of the lower leg, ankle and foot may be the result of tibialis posterior tendinitis. The tibialis posterior tendon stabilizes the foot against eversion and supports the medial arch of the foot, which puts friction and tension on the tendon. If the arch falls, stress on the tendon will increase. This can occur with poor running mechanics, improper footwear or untreated injuries.

Cause of injury
Improper running mechanics. Improper footwear. Prior injury to the medial side of the ankle.

Signs and symptoms
Pain and tenderness over the inner side of the shin, ankle and foot. Pain when walking or running. Some swelling may be noted over the tendon.

Complications if left unattended
If left unattended, this condition can lead to a fallen arch or a complete rupture of the tendon. The pain may cause a change in footfall during running leading to injuries in other structures of the foot and ankle.

Immediate treatment
RICER. Anti-inflammatory medication.

Rehabilitation and prevention
After pain subsides it is important to stretch and strengthen the calf muscles to support the tendon and speed recovery. Arch supports may be required until the tendon heals and the muscles are strengthened. Gradual reintroduction into activity is important and proper warm-ups will help prevent a recurrence of the injury. Proper footwear and corrections of any mechanical inefficiency will also help prevent this injury.

Long-term prognosis
Proper treatment should lead to a complete recovery. The longer the condition exists before treatment the longer recovery will take. In some cases orthotics may be required to prevent a recurrence.

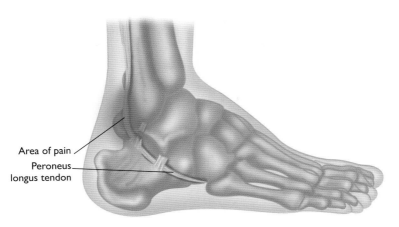

Area of pain

Peroneus longus tendon

PERONEAL TENDON SUBLUXATION

The tendons of peroneus longus and peroneus brevis run from the peroneal muscles in the lateral calf to the foot. They pass around the lateral malleolus through a groove in the bone. Peroneal tendon subluxation (dislocation) is most commonly a chronic condition that develops after a sprain or fracture. The tendon moves out of the groove in which it runs due to damage to the ligamentous structures designed to hold it in place. Pain on the lateral ankle and a popping sensation are possible signs of this condition.

Running and jumping can cause repetitive stress to the tendon especially when it is subluxating repeatedly. Some people are predisposed to this injury due to a shallow, or non-existent groove where the tendons lie. Peroneal tendon subluxation may also occur if the tip of the lateral malleolus is fractured by forced dorsiflexion or a direct blow.

Cause of injury

Tearing or stretching of the ligaments that support the tendons, usually due to an ankle sprain or fracture. Repetitive stress to the tendons, causing inflammation and swelling, allowing the tendons to slide out of the groove.

Signs and symptoms

Pain and tenderness along the tendons. Popping or snapping sensation on the lateral side of the ankle. Swelling may be noted along the bottom of the fibula.

Complications if left unattended

The peroneal tendons become irritated when they dislocate, which causes inflammation. This inflammation can lead to tearing or complete rupture of the tendons if left untreated.

Immediate treatment

RICER. Anti-inflammatory medication. Possible immobilization, especially with acute dislocation.

Rehabilitation and prevention

Strengthening of the muscles in the lower leg after pain subsides and normal function returns will help support the tendons. Treating ankle sprains properly will help prevent subluxation. Strong calf and shin muscles will help support the whole foot and ankle structure, preventing this condition as well.

Long-term prognosis

When treated promptly, subluxation of the peroneal tendons usually responds well to non-surgical techniques. In some cases, surgery may be required to repair the sheath and ligaments that cover the tendon to restore stability.

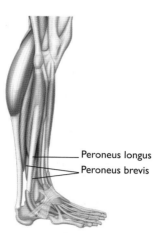

Peroneus longus
Peroneus brevis

PERONEAL TENDINITIS

The tendons of peroneus longus and peroneus brevis run from the peroneal muscles in the lateral calf to the foot. The peroneal muscles are involved in stabilizing the foot and providing support to the ankle to prevent lateral rolling of the joint. Peroneal tendinitis is most commonly a result of overuse of the peroneal muscles or of inversion sprains which stretch the peroneal tendons. It can be caused by excessive pronation of the foot as the peroneal muscles have to work harder to stabilize the foot when it is pronated.

Running and jumping involve repeated contraction of the peroneal muscles and can lead to inflammation of their tendons. Runners who often run on uneven surfaces or have excessive pronation often develop peroneal tendinitis.

Cause of injury
Over-pronation of the foot during running or jumping. Prior ankle injury leading to an incorrect path of travel for the tendons.

Signs and symptoms
Pain and tenderness along the tendons. Pain is most severe at the beginning of the activity and diminishes as the activity continues. Gradual increase in pain over time.

Complications if left unattended
Unattended tendinitis can lead to a complete rupture of the tendons. Peroneal tendinitis can lead to subluxations. The chronic inflammation can also lead to damage to the ligaments surrounding the tendons.

Immediate treatment
Rest, especially from running or jumping activities. Ice. Anti-inflammatory medication.

Rehabilitation and prevention
Stretching of the calf muscles and a gradual reintroduction into activity is important for rehabilitation. During the recovery period it is important to identify and correct any foot or gait abnormalities that may be contributing to the problem. Prevention of this condition requires strong, flexible muscles of the lower leg to support the foot and ankle.

Long-term prognosis
With proper treatment, peroneal tendinitis will usually heal completely with no lingering effects. In rare cases the tendinitis may not respond to traditional treatment and may require surgical intervention to relieve the pressure causing the inflammation. Orthotics to support the medial arch may be required in some cases.

OSTEOCHONDRITIS DISSECANS

Osteochondritis dissecans occurs when a fragment of bone adjacent to the articular surface of a joint is deprived of its blood supply, leading to avascular necrosis. Fractures can occur on the surface of the talus or the cartilage may become bruised from any twisting injury causing the talus to come into hard contact with the tibia or fibula. The poor blood supply of articular cartilage means that repairing damage is difficult for the body. Damaged cartilage becomes brittle and pieces, or loose bodies, may break off. Loose cartilage in the joint can cause pain and inflammation.

The space in the ankle joint is very small and when a bone or cartilage fragment from the talus gets lodged in the joint cavity it can cause pain, swelling and loss of movement in the ankle. These symptoms may come and go as the free-floating fragment floats in and out of the joint cavity. Prior ankle injuries make a person susceptible to this condition, as does any compromise of the blood supply to the feet.

Cause of injury
Loss of blood flow to the articular surface of the talus along with injury to the bone. Repetitive wear on the cartilage and bone surface of the talus. Previous ankle injury.

Signs and symptoms
Pain and discomfort in the joint. If the fragment becomes detached and lodged in the joint, swelling and loss of movement may occur. A catching sensation in the ankle may be felt.

Complications if left unattended
Loose bodies in the joint can cause scarring and additional damage if left unattended. As the joint moves and the loose body grinds against the cartilage and bone surfaces, it will wear at these surfaces making them rough and eventually lead to arthritis.

Immediate treatment
Anti-inflammatory medication. Rest and possible immobilization of the joint. Referral to a sports medicine professional.

Rehabilitation and prevention
Rehabilitating the ankle after this type of injury includes strengthening the muscles of the lower leg to offer additional support to the joint. Stretching and range of motion activities may be required if the ankle was immobilized for treatment. Gradual return to activity will help to prevent it from recurring immediately. Treating all ankle injuries properly, no matter how minor, will help maintain a good blood supply to the joint and protect the talus.

Long-term prognosis
Many times the loose body does not completely detach from the bone allowing the body to reabsorb it. If a loose body does become detached it may require surgical removal. If allowed to wear at the joint loose bodies can lead to osteoarthritis especially in the older athlete.

104: SUPINATION

SUPINATION

Supination occurs at the subtalar joint between the talus and the calcaneus (heel bone). The distal (lower) ends of the tibia and fibula rest on the talus of the foot at the talocrural joint. This is traditionally referred to as a hinge joint because its main function is to allow flexion and extension of the ankle. The subtalar joint below allows pronation and supination of the foot. Pronation and supination movements aid balance and improve shock absorption.

Supination is the outward rolling of the foot at the ankle. This is a normal movement during the push-off phase of running, walking or jumping. Excessive supination can cause damage to the lateral ligaments, tendons and muscles of the lower leg and ankle. Acute over-supination may cause stretching or tearing of the lateral ligaments of the foot and ankle. Excessive supination can lead to a weakening of the ankle structure and decreased stability.

Cause of injury
Weak or loose tendons and ligaments in the ankle. Weak or fatigued muscles of the lower leg. Forceful outward rolling of the ankle. Improper or worn footwear. Uneven or sloped running (or landing) surface.

Signs and symptoms
Pain in the arch, heel and/or knees and hips. Instability in the ankle. Pain over the outside of the ankle. Pain may be immediate with acute over-supination (such as an ankle sprain).

Complications if left unattended
May lead to chronic weakness and instability in the ankle. The pain and improper gait may lead to compensation and injury to other structures and tissues. The ligaments may lose their elasticity from excessive stretching and tearing may occur.

Immediate treatment
Rest, ice and anti-inflammatory/analgesic medication. Acute over-supination may require medical attention and immobilization. Chronic supination will require correction of the underlying problems whilst allowing adequate rest for the tissues to recover.

Rehabilitation and prevention
Proper warm-up is essential. Strengthening and stretching of the muscles of the lower leg may help support the ankle, keep it moving in the correct plane and reduce excessive supination. Orthotics and gait analysis may be required. Gradual return to full activity is recommended and retraining of the athlete to improve or correct running form is important. Ensure proper footwear and a smooth, flat running (or landing) surface.

Long-term prognosis
Will respond well if treated early with a good rehabilitation plan. The length of time the condition is allowed to persist will also affect the recovery time. In rare cases, surgery may be required to tighten the tendons or correct skeletal factors.

PRONATION

Pronation occurs at the subtalar joint between the talus and the calcaneus (heel bone). The distal (lower) ends of the tibia and fibula rest on the talus of the foot at the talocrural joint. This is traditionally referred to as a hinge joint because its main function is to allow flexion and extension of the ankle. The subtalar joint below allows pronation and supination of the foot. Pronation and supination movements aid balance and improve shock absorption.

Pronation is the inward rolling of the foot at the ankle during walking or running. While some pronation is natural and part of normal gait, excessive pronation can lead to chronic injuries and acute over-pronation can lead to strains or sprains.

The strong medial ligaments of the ankle help provide support and prevent excessive pronation. The tibialis anterior and posterior muscles of the lower leg also offer support. When ligaments are loose or the muscles fatigue the support is lost which results in more pronation. This causes the arch of the foot to flatten out which in turn further stretches the ligaments. During weightbearing in the mid-stance phase of the gait cycle there is a tendency for the calcaneus to evert (roll in) and the forefoot to abduct (point outward) as the ankle moves into dorsiflexion.

Cause of injury
Loose or torn tendons from previous ankle injuries. Weak or fatigued muscles of the lower leg. Improper or worn footwear. Uneven running (or landing) surfaces.

Signs and symptoms
Pain in the arch, heel and/or knees and hips. Pain during the landing phase of running or jumping. Visible inward rolling of the foot and ankle. Instability in the ankle. Pain may be immediate for acute over-pronation, such as an ankle eversion sprain, or gradual for chronic pronation disorders.

Complications if left unattended
Pronation has been linked with shin splints, plantar fasciitis, chondromalacia patellae, tendinitis and even stress fractures. The longer pronation continues the more the medial ligaments of the foot and ankle will be stretched, leading to ankle instability. The arches may flatten out and lead to other problems of the foot. Chronic pronation of the foot beyond normal ranges can lead to overuse and chronic injuries.

Immediate treatment
Rest, ice and anti-inflammatory/analgesic medication. For acute injuries, immobilization and reduction of weightbearing activities may be required. For chronic injuries seek the help of a qualified sports medicine specialist to help identify and correct the problem.

Rehabilitation and prevention
Correct the underlying problem, e.g. if due to the running surface change the surface to one that is flat or smooth. If due to footwear try new or different shoes. If necessary use orthotics and gait training. Warm-up properly. Stretching and strengthening will offer support and keep the muscles of the lower leg strong and flexible. Completely rehabilitate any ankle injury before returning to sport to prevent recurrence.

Long-term prognosis
The condition usually responds well to treatment, although the longer pronation goes untreated and is allowed to cause damage to the ligaments the longer the recovery time. In very rare cases, surgical intervention may be required to correct any underlying orthopedic issues.

REHABILITATION EXERCISES

Calf raise

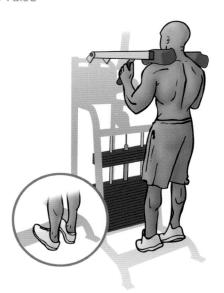

Stand upright and place your toes on the edge of the step and your shoulders securely under the padded weight. Slowly raise the weight up by straightening your ankles, then lower the weight to the start position and repeat.

Single-legged calf raise

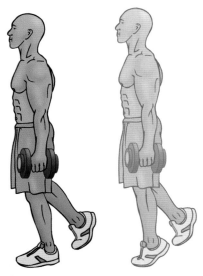

With a dumbbell in each hand raise one leg slightly off the ground. Slowly raise up by straightening your ankle, then lower yourself to the start position, repeat, and then switch sides.

Ankle jumps

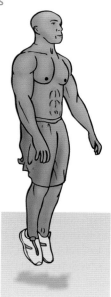

With your arms at your sides, jump off the ground using only your ankles and calves.

Goose-steps

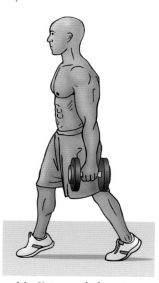

With a dumbbell in each hand, take 10 steps forward walking only on your toes.

Achilles stretch

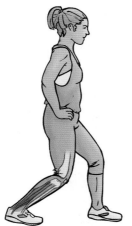

Stand upright and take one big step backward.
Bend your back leg and push your heel toward
the ground.

Cross-over shin stretch

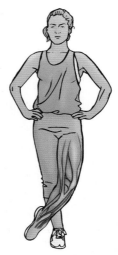

Stand upright and place the top of your toes on
the ground in front of your other foot. Slowly
bend your other leg to force your ankle to the
ground.

Sports Injuries of the Foot

ANATOMY AND PHYSIOLOGY

The foot consists of twenty-six small bones. The seven tarsals form the ankle. The two largest tarsals carry the body weight: the calcaneus, or the heel bone, and the talus. The talus sits between the tibia, the fibula and the calcaneus. The tibia and fibula rest on top of the talus which rests on the calcaneus. The other tarsal bones are: the navicular, medial cuneiform, intermediate cuneiform, lateral cuneiform and the cuboid. The five metatarsals are long, narrow bones that form the instep or sole of the foot and the fourteen phalanges consist of short, narrow bones that form the toes, with two joints in the big toe and three in the others.

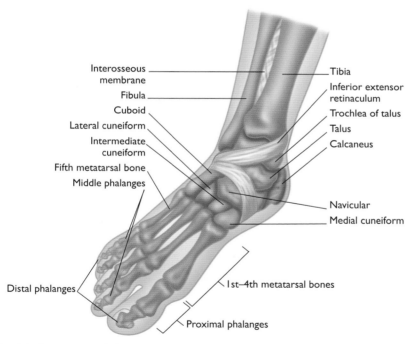

Labels (left side): Interosseous membrane, Fibula, Cuboid, Lateral cuneiform, Intermediate cuneiform, Fifth metatarsal bone, Middle phalanges, Distal phalanges, 1st–4th metatarsal bones, Proximal phalanges

Labels (right side): Tibia, Inferior extensor retinaculum, Trochlea of talus, Talus, Calcaneus, Navicular, Medial cuneiform

The bones of the right foot, anteromedial view.

The sesamoid bones of the foot are located on the plantar surface of the first metatarsal head. The sesamoid bones are spherical and embedded in the tendon of the flexor hallucis brevis (FHB). They reduce friction and guide the tendon to aid transmission of the force generated by FHB which is responsible for 'toeing off' in walking and running. The sesamoid bones also help elevate the bones of the big toe and assist in weightbearing.

The sheer number of articulations between the bones of the foot mean they are usually described in groups: the subtalar joint (between the talus and calcaneus); transverse tarsal joints (the articulations between the talus, navicular, cuboid and the cuneiforms); tarsometatarsal joints (the articulations between the cuneiforms, the cuboid and the metatarsals); metatarsophalangeal joints and interphalangeal joints.

In addition to the ligaments stabilizing the many joints between adjacent bones of the foot, strong ligaments criss-cross the plantar surface (the sole of the foot). Bands of fascia known as retinacula keep the tendons of the muscles of the feet and lower leg in place around the ankle.

The plantar fascia is a thick, tough, collagenous sheet of ligament on the plantar surface which stretches from the calcaneus to the proximal phalanges. It provides cushioning and structural support to the foot and the arches, and acts as a point of attachment for the many muscles of the foot.

The foot is not a rigid structure. The bones of the foot flatten on weightbearing and the foot pronates and supinates during gait. This dynamic flexibility is supported by medial and lateral longitudinal arches and two transverse arches under the tarsal and metatarsal bones. Arches are formed by the shape of the bones of the foot and are strengthened by strong ligaments (the spring ligament of the medial arch is one of the most clinically important) and by the muscles of the foot and the lower leg.

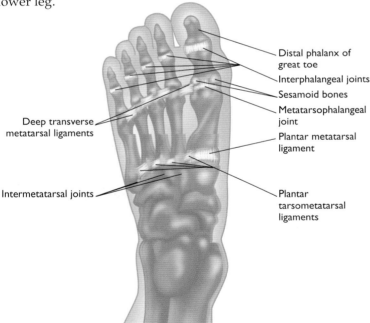

The bones of the right foot, plantar view.

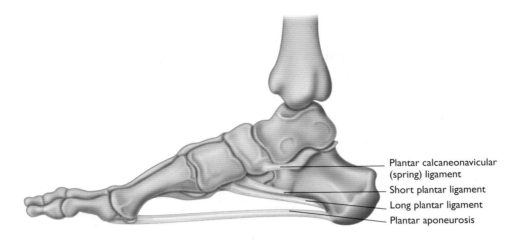

A multitude of muscles control the foot. Some of these originate in the lower leg. Others, the intrinsic muscles of the foot, originate in the foot itself. Along with the structure of the joints, this allows for a wide range of movement at the foot and ankle. These include flexion and extension (plantarflexion) at the ankle and at the individual joints of the toes; eversion and inversion occur at the subtalar articulation between the calcaneus and talus; the whole foot may be adducted and abducted away from the midline of the body and the toes themselves may be spread or pulled together. Conjoint movements over several joints allow rotation of the foot on the ankle and pronation and supination.

Extensor hallucis longus (EHL) and extensor digitorum longus (EDL) are the main extensor muscles of the toes. Their tendons run over the front of the ankle and foot and attach to the phalanxes of the toes. These muscles dorsiflex the foot and work in opposition to the flexor muscles. The flexor group of muscles, flexor hallucis longus (FHL) and flexor digitorum longus (FDL), have tendons that run behind the medial malleolus of the ankle and under the foot, attaching to the toes. These muscles plantarflex the foot and toes.

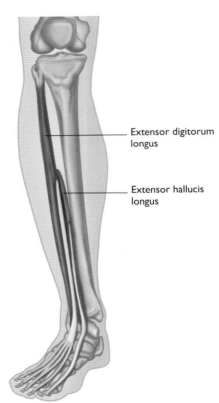

The main extensor muscles of the toes.

There are four layers of muscle in the sole of the foot. The first layer is the most inferior (the most superficial and closest to the ground on weightbearing) and comprises abductor hallucis, flexor digitorum brevis and abductor digiti minimi. Abductor digiti minimi forms the lateral margin of the sole of the foot. The second layer contains the lumbricales and quadratus plantae, plus the tendons of flexor hallucis longus and flexor digitorum longus. The third layer contains flexor hallucis brevis, adductor hallucis and flexor digiti minimi brevis. The fourth layer is the deepest and consists of the four dorsal interossei, the three plantar interossei and the tendons of tibialis posterior and peroneus longus.

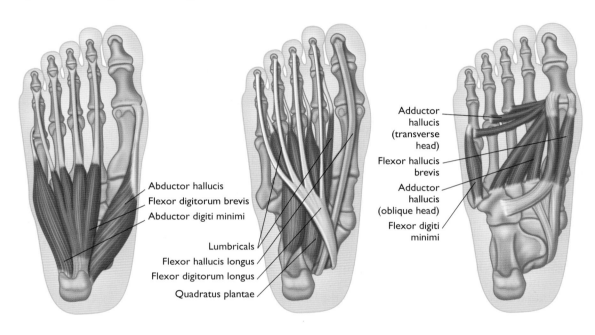

Muscles associated with movement of the ankle and foot.

FRACTURE OF THE FOOT

A foot fracture may involve any of the 26 bones of the foot but most commonly occurs to the metatarsals when direct force is applied to the shaft. Contact sports and sports that could result in high-impact landings or collisions have a higher rate of foot fractures. Those athletes with lower bone density due to nutritional deficiency, osteoporosis (or absent menstrual cycles in female athletes) are more susceptible to fractures.

Cause of injury
Trauma to the bones of the foot, e.g. fall, blow, collision or violent twisting.

Signs and symptoms
Pain, which can be severe. Swelling and discolouration. Possible deformity at the fracture site. Pain on weightbearing and possible inability to walk. Numbness of the foot or toes.

Complications if left unattended
A fracture that is left untreated can lead to damage to the blood vessels and nerves in and around the fracture site. The bones may heal incorrectly or not heal at all. Weakness and instability in the foot may result.

Immediate treatment
Immediate removal from activity. Ice, elevation and possible immobilization. Seek immediate medical treatment.

Rehabilitation and prevention
After pain subsides, stretching of the muscles that were not used during recovery is important. Strengthening of muscles that have atrophied due to lack of use during immobilization is a must. Strong muscles to support the foot are essential to prevent foot fractures. Avoiding direct trauma to the foot is the best tool for prevention. Proper footwear to offer support and protection will also help prevent this injury.

Long-term prognosis
If allowed to heal completely, a fracture will usually heal to become stronger than before the injury. In fractures that are compound or misaligned, surgical pinning may be required to stabilize the bone until it heals. If the ligaments are stretched or torn the chance of re-injury increases.

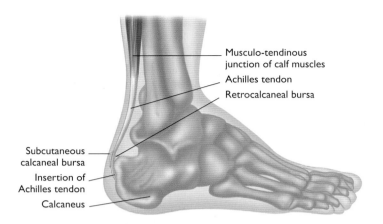

Musculo-tendinous junction of calf muscles
Achilles tendon
Retrocalcaneal bursa
Subcutaneous calcaneal bursa
Insertion of Achilles tendon
Calcaneus

RETROCALCANEAL BURSITIS

The retrocalcaneal bursa lies between the Achilles tendon insertion and the calcaneus (heel bone) and helps to lubricate and cushion the tendon as it runs over the heel. This bursa is stressed during repetitive movements of the ankle and foot such as during running, walking or jumping. The repetitive friction of the tendon running over the bursa during forceful plantarflexion during push-off compresses the bursa between the tendon and bone and can cause inflammation.

Worn or incorrectly sized footwear or excessive pronation of the foot can lead to problems with this bursa and the Achilles tendon. Shoes that fit too tightly, especially around the heel, may put additional stress on the tendon and bursa.

Cause of injury
Repetitive stress to the bursa by the friction of the Achilles tendon during walking, running or jumping. Increasing duration or distance too quickly. Improper footwear. Gait dysfunction such as over-pronation. Injury to the Achilles tendon.

Signs and symptoms
Pain, especially with walking, running or jumping. Tenderness over the heel area. Redness and slight swelling may be noted over the heel.

Complications if left unattended
The bursa can rupture completely if the injury is left unattended. This complete rupture could lead to other problems with the Achilles tendon due to increased friction. The pain may make it difficult to rise up onto the toes during walking, running or jumping.

Immediate treatment
Rest from activities that cause pain. Ice. Anti-inflammatory medication.

Rehabilitation and prevention
Strengthening the muscles of the calf and stretching the muscles of the lower leg will facilitate healing. Using activities that do not irritate the area to maintain fitness levels is essential. Keeping the muscles strong and flexible and allowing adequate warm-up before all activities will help prevent bursitis.

Long-term prognosis
Proper treatment and rest should lead to a complete recovery. In rare cases the fluid that builds up due to the inflammation may need to be drained to facilitate healing. Surgery is only necessary in extreme cases that do not respond to rest and rehabilitation.

STRESS FRACTURE

Stress fractures in the foot are usually a result of repetitive impact to the bones of the feet. Running or jumping on hard surfaces, changing the duration or distance of workouts too quickly or fatigued muscles that can no longer absorb shock can lead to the formation of small cracks in the bone. The small cracks accumulate and become a stress fracture.

A stress fracture can occur in any of the bones of the foot but are generally seen in the metatarsals. The calcaneus can also become fractured due to improper footwear or as a result of an old injury that has gone untreated. A weak point in the bone from a previous injury or due to bone remodelling can develop stress fractures under normal stress conditions.

Cause of injury
Repetitive trauma to the bones of the foot. Weakened area of bone due to previous injury or other condition. Muscle fatigue making the muscles ineffective shock absorbers.

Signs and symptoms
Pain at the site of the fracture. Pain on weightbearing, with inability to walk in severe cases. Swelling may be noted over the fracture site. Some loss of foot function may be noted.

Complications if left unattended
More serious stress fracture including a complete break in the bone may occur if left unattended. Swelling and inflammation may cause circulatory and nerve problems in the foot. Pain may increase to the point of disability and inability to walk.

Immediate treatment
RICER. Anti-inflammatory medication.

Rehabilitation and prevention
Strengthening the muscles that support the foot will help to lessen the impact of bodyweight and ground impact forces on the foot. A gradual return to activity after the injury has healed is important to prevent recurrence. Proper footwear, correct warm-up techniques, avoiding hard running surfaces and a calcium-rich diet will help prevent stress fractures in the foot.

Long-term prognosis
Stress fractures will usually heal completely and have no lingering effects if rest and rehabilitation are used. The fracture site should heal to become stronger than it was originally. Only in severe cases where the bone fractures completely and does not respond to rest and immobilization will surgery be required.

EXTENSOR AND FLEXOR TENDINITIS

The tendons of the muscles responsible for flexing and extending the toes and foot can become inflamed and irritated. Overuse, tightness in opposing muscles and/or the calf muscles, joint dysfunction or gait abnormalities can cause this condition. Extensor tendinitis is more common but flexor tendinitis tends to be more painful and debilitating. Dancers are most commonly associated with injury to the flexor tendons.

Cause of injury
Extensor tendinitis: Tight calf muscles, over-exertion of the extensor muscles, fallen arches.
Flexor tendinitis: Repetitive stress to the tendon from excessive dorsiflexion (extension) of the foot.

Signs and symptoms
Extensor tendinitis: Pain on the top of the foot, pain when dorsiflexing the toes, some strength loss may be experienced.
Flexor tendinitis: Pain along the course of the tendon, in the medial arch of the foot and behind the medial malleolus of the ankle. Pain when walking or flexing the toes against resistance.

Complications if left unattended
Tendinitis when left unattended can cause strains to the associated muscles and could lead to a complete rupture of the tendon. The pain may become severe enough to limit all activity.

Immediate treatment
Rest from activities that cause pain. Ice the tendon. Anti-inflammatory medication.

Rehabilitation and prevention
While resting the foot it is important to identify the conditions that caused the problem. Stretching the calf muscles and tibialis anterior on the shin will help relieve the pressure on the tendons. Warming-up and gradually increasing workload will help prevent tendinitis. Orthotics may be required when returning to activity to correct any arch problems.

Long-term prognosis
Most people recover completely from tendinitis with simple rest and correction of the cause(s). In some rare cases surgery may be required to reduce the pressure on the tendons and relieve the inflammation.

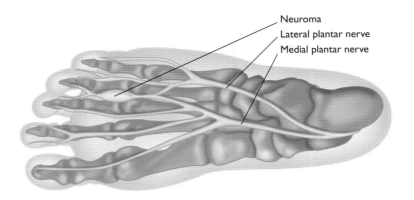

Neuroma
Lateral plantar nerve
Medial plantar nerve

MORTON'S NEUROMA

Branches of the plantar nerve supply the toes and run between the metatarsal heads where they can become compressed, which causes inflammation and swelling. Morton's neuroma is caused by swelling of nerve and scar tissue causing compression of the plantar nerve. It is characterized by pain, burning sensations and/or numbness on the plantar surface of the foot, usually between the third and fourth metatarsals.

Running (especially sprinting), walking and jumping all place repetitive stress on the metatarsals and have the potential to cause Morton's neuroma. Foot deformities, underlying gait abnormalities such as over-pronation or tight-fitting shoes which compress the foot can also lead to this condition.

Cause of injury
Repetitive stress or trauma to the ball of the foot, such as with running, walking or jumping. Pronation. Wearing footwear that compresses the foot. Injuries to the metatarsals of the third and fourth toes.

Signs and symptoms
Pain and/or burning sensation in the affected area. Possible loss of sensation in the third and fourth toes. Possible numbness, tingling or cramping in the forefoot. While weightbearing in shoes, severe pain on the lateral side of the foot may be present which is relieved by going barefoot.

Complications if left unattended
If left unattended a neuroma may lead to permanent nerve damage. Permanent loss of sensation to the toes may result. Pain will increase without treatment eventually leading to disability.

Immediate treatment
Rest from or modification of activity. Anti-inflammatory medication. Ice.

Rehabilitation and prevention
A gradual return to activity and avoiding repetitive trauma to the forefoot will help speed recovery. Padding may be needed when activity is resumed. The most important step in prevention of this condition is to use footwear that allows plenty of room for the forefoot. Narrow-toed shoes and high heels should be avoided.

Long-term prognosis
When treated properly a neuroma should recover completely without any long-term effects. The longer the injury goes untreated the higher the potential for lingering effects. Surgery may be required if conservative treatment does not lead to recovery.

111: SESAMOIDITIS

SESAMOIDITIS

The sesamoid bones in the tendon of flexor hallucis brevis on the base of the head of the first metatarsal can become injured and inflamed causing a condition similar to tendinitis. Runners, dancers and catchers in baseball are all susceptible to this injury. Increasing activity too quickly causes additional trauma to the small sesamoid bones.

Cause of injury
Increased activity without proper conditioning. Little natural padding in the forefoot leaving the sesamoid bones unprotected. High arches leading to running on the balls of the feet.

Signs and symptoms
Gradual onset of pain. Pain over the bone and surrounding tendon. Pain increases with activity.

Complications if left unattended
If left unattended this condition can worsen to the point that the pain becomes debilitating. Inflammation in the tendon can cause irritation to surrounding tissue. As with tendinitis, a complete rupture may occur if the condition is allowed to go untreated.

Immediate treatment
Rest. Ice. Anti-inflammatory medication.

Rehabilitation and prevention
Finding activities that do not stress or irritate the injured area will help to maintain fitness levels while healing takes place. Strengthening the muscles of the lower leg will help support the foot. Wearing padding inside the shoes may be necessary when returning to activity. Gradually increasing distance or duration will help prevent this condition, as will warming-up properly before beginning exercise. Orthotics or implants to correct arch problems may also help prevent sesamoiditis.

Long-term prognosis
Sesamoiditis responds well to rest and anti-inflammatory treatments. Complete recovery can be expected with no lingering effects. In rare cases where the condition does not respond to preliminary treatments surgical intervention may be required.

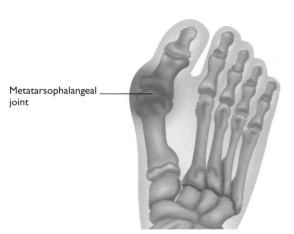

Metatarsophalangeal joint

BUNIONS

Tight or ill-fitting shoes can lead to swelling and enlargement of the base of the big toe known as a bunion. Injury to the big toe, abnormal stress on the outside of the toe and reduced force transference through the foot during gait due to medial arch problems can also lead to bunions. Women are much more likely to get bunions than men due to the wearing of tighter-fitting shoes. A bunion-like condition may develop on the lateral aspect of the fifth toe called a bunionette.

Bunions are typically found on the medial aspect of the metatarsophalangeal joint which connects the toe and foot. When tight-fitting shoes, an injury or other condition causes pressure on the toe (forcing it inward) the joint becomes inflamed and enlarged. There is inflammation of the bursa overlying the medial aspect of the first metatarsal head. The first metatarsal moves medially while the toe moves laterally toward the second toe, sometimes even sliding under it, forming a hallux valgus deformity.

Cause of injury
Tight-fitting shoes. Untreated injury to the big toe. Unusual pressure to the outside of the first toe. Over-pronation of the foot.

Signs and symptoms
Bump at the base of the big toe. Hallux valgus deformity. Redness and tenderness in the affected area. Pain on walking.

Complications if left unattended
Bunions left unattended may lead to further complications such as bursitis, difficulty walking, arthritis and chronic pain. Hallux valgus deformities may cause further problems due to misalignment.

Immediate treatment
Remove and discard tight-fitting shoes. Wear roomier shoes especially when exercising. Padding the bunion may relieve some of the pain. Anti-inflammatory medication.

Rehabilitation and prevention
Prevention is essential when assessing bunions. Footwear with enough room for the feet will help prevent this condition. Avoiding undue pressure and taking care to treat even minor toe injuries will also prevent bunions. Padding the area when exercising will help alleviate pain.

Long-term prognosis
Bunions respond reasonably well to treatment. In cases where the bunion does not respond to treatment and function is significantly compromised, surgery may be needed to correct the condition. Depending on the surgical procedure recovery may be almost immediate or require several months.

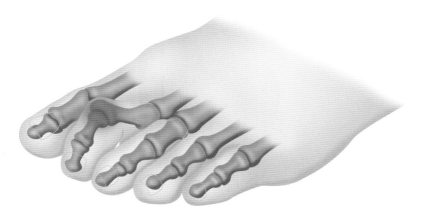

HAMMER TOE

Hammer toe gets its name from the hammer- or claw-like appearance of the affected toe. The proximal phalanx (most often that of the second toe) is hyperextended (dorsiflexed) at the metatarsophalangeal joint while the middle phalanx is strongly flexed at the proximal interphalangeal joint. The distal phalanx may also be hyperextended. This puts increased pressure on the ball of the foot and causes the top of the middle phalanx to rub against the shoe. Corns and/or calluses may develop due to the pressure of the toe against the shoes.

Ill-fitting shoes may cause this condition. Weakness in the intrinsic muscles of the foot or nerve damage to the toe flexor muscles may also result in this condition. Diabetes, stroke, arthritis or prior injury can also cause a dysfunctional flexion of the toes.

Cause of injury
Ill-fitting shoes. Muscle or nerve damage to the toe flexor muscles.

Signs and symptoms
Hammer-like appearance of the toe. Pain and difficulty moving the toe. Corns and calluses may develop on the affected toe.

Complications if left unattended
When left unattended hammer toe can lead to other problems such as arthritis, painful corns and calluses and flexor tendinitis. It may also lead to a complete inability to extend or straighten the toe.

Immediate treatment
Switch to roomier shoes. Anti-inflammatory medication.

Rehabilitation and prevention
Stretching and strengthening the toes will aid recovery and correct the alignment of the toes if they are still flexible. Selecting properly fitted shoes and stretching the toes regularly will help prevent hammer toe from developing. Straps and padding may be required to relieve some of the pain.

Long-term prognosis
Surgery may be required if the toe has become inflexible and other treatments do not work.

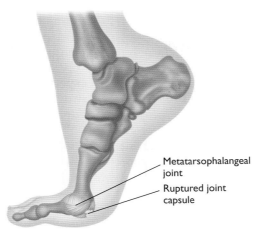

Metatarsophalangeal joint

Ruptured joint capsule

TURF TOE

Pain at the base of the big toe may be a result of turf toe. Athletes who jam their toe or repeatedly push off when running or jumping are susceptible to this injury. Turf toe is often caused by forced hyperextension of the metatarsophalangeal joint. The name turf toe comes from the fact that this injury is common among athletes who play on artificial turf.

Turf toe develops at the metatarsophalangeal joint at the base of the great toe. The plantar joint capsule or ligament is torn leading to instability and pain. This can lead to dislocations, cartilage wear and eventually arthritis. The tendons that cross the joint can become involved as well. Jamming the toe, or pushing off when running or jumping puts stress on the capsule and can lead to tearing.

Cause of injury
Jamming the toe. Repeated pushing off on the toe, especially on a harder surface such as artificial turf.

Signs and symptoms
Pain at the base of the toe. Some swelling may be noted in the joint. Pain increases when pushing off with the toe.

Complications if left unattended
Turf toe can lead to chronic pain and the inability to run or jump. When left unattended turf toe can lead to other conditions such as toe dislocations and arthritis.

Immediate treatment
Rest. Ice. Anti-inflammatory medication.

Rehabilitation and prevention
As the pain subsides it is important to work on the strength and flexibility of the toes. Adjusting the way pressure is applied to the foot when pushing off will also help to correct the condition(s) that caused the turf toe. Alternating workouts between hard and softer surfaces will help prevent the development of this condition. Special inserts that support the toe may be used when returning to activity. A gradual return to full activity is important.

Long-term prognosis
Turf toe does have a tendency to return when working out on the same surface. In most cases pain will subside and normal function will return. In very rare cases surgery is required to alleviate the symptoms.

PES PLANUS (FLAT FEET)

Pes planus (flat feet or fallen arches) is a condition in which the foot flattens and the medial longtitudinal arch falls toward the ground. People with flat feet often have difficulty finding shoes that fit properly which can lead to other foot problems or gait disturbances. This condition is the opposite of claw foot (pes cavus) but is much more common.

In pes planus, the flattening of the arch is associated with over-pronation, the excessive inward rolling of the foot and ankle, which often leads to other injuries of the foot, ankle, knees, hips and lower back. The low arch puts additional stress on the calf muscles and the medial ankle and is a possible contributor to ankle sprain and shin splints. Athletes with pes planus must work to maximize strength in the arch and the affected muscles.

Cause of injury
Weakness or instability in the muscles, tendons and ligaments in the lower leg and arch of the foot. May be hereditary or acquired due to trauma or illness.

Signs and symptoms
Unusually low, flattened arch in which the entire sole of the foot makes contact with the ground. Pain in the foot, ankle and lower leg, especially when walking, running or when standing for long periods of time.

Complications if left unattended
Most people with flat feet don't experience pain or any other problems but athletes or very active individuals with pes planus can experience pain and possible injury to other structures in the foot, ankle and lower leg. Bunions.

Immediate treatment
If pain is experienced, rest and limiting weightbearing activities will usually bring quick relief. If pain continues see a sports medicine professional or podiatrist for a complete foot and gait analysis.

Rehabilitation and prevention
Strength exercises for the ankle, feet and toes are the first and most important step in rehabilitation. Foot gymnastics (games and exercises for the feet and toes) and barefoot walking on sand or other uneven surfaces will help to strengthen all the soft tissues of the foot and lower leg. Finding properly fitting shoes, orthotics, arch supports or custom made shoes is important for comfort, to help support the arch and prevent injury due to instability of the foot.

Long term prognosis
When treated properly, much of the pain associated with pes planus can be relieved. Surgery may be a last resort, especially when pain is severe and other treatments do not help.

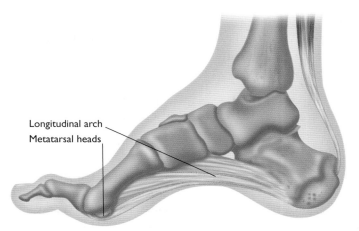

Longitudinal arch
Metatarsal heads

PES CAVUS (CLAW FOOT)

Pes cavus (claw foot) is a condition that gives the foot a claw-like appearance. People with claw foot often have difficulty finding shoes that fit properly which can lead to other foot problems or gait disturbances. This condition is the opposite of flat feet (pes planus) but is much less common.

In pes cavus, the exaggerated height and inflexibility of the longitudinal arch is associated with tight calf muscles, increased stress on the Achilles tendon and pain in the forefoot as foot positioning puts additional stress on the metatarsal heads. The high arch puts additional stress on the calf muscles and the lateral ankle. Athletes with pes cavus must work to maximize flexibility in the arch and the affected muscles or work around it in their activities.

Cause of injury
May be inherited or acquired due to trauma or neurological disease. Possibly secondary to contractures or disturbed balance of the muscles.

Signs and symptoms
Unusually high, inflexible arch. Pain in the foot, especially when walking or running. Toes may be bent.

Complications if left unattended
Pes cavus can cause chronic pain and possible injury to other structures in the foot. Foot and ankle instability is common and could lead to strains and sprains.

Immediate treatment
Stretch the calf muscles and the foot. Contact a sports medicine professional if painful and unresponsive to self-management.

Rehabilitation and prevention
Stretching the calf muscles and the foot is the first and most important step in rehabilitation. Finding properly fitting shoes is important for comfort, to help support the arch and prevent injury due to instability of the foot. Strengthening the muscles of the lower leg will also support the foot. If surgery is required it will be important to increase strength and flexibility in the muscles that are immobilized.

Long-term prognosis
When treated properly, much of the pain associated with claw foot can be relieved. Surgery may be an option especially when pain is severe and other treatments do not help.

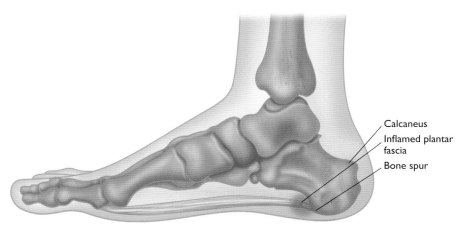

Calcaneus

Inflamed plantar fascia

Bone spur

PLANTAR FASCIITIS

Plantar fasciitis is an overuse condition affecting the plantar fascia or aponeurosis at its insertion on the calcaneus. The plantar fascia is a tough, fibrous sheet which runs from the tuberosity of the calcaneus to the metatarsal heads. It is important for supporting the longitudinal arch of the foot, as a point of muscle attachment and for cushioning the bones of the foot.

Repetitive ankle movement, especially when restricted by tight calves, can irritate the plantar fascia at the calcaneus. Pain is usually felt in the heel especially upon rising from an extended rest. Walking or running, especially on hard surfaces and with tight calf muscles, makes an athlete more susceptible to this injury. High or fallen arches and incorrect footwear can also lead to plantar fasciitis.

Cause of injury
Running on hard surfaces. Improper or ill-fitting footwear. Arch problems. Training errors. Overuse. Over-pronation. Poor flexibility of the calf muscles (gastrocnemius, soleus and plantaris) and Achilles tendon.

Signs and symptoms
Pain under the heel which is worse after exercise or when rising from an extended rest. Pain may diminish during exercise but return after the activity is stopped.

Complications if left unattended
Plantar fasciitis that is left unattended can lead to chronic pain that may cause a change in walking or running gait. This in turn can lead to knee, hip and lower back problems.

Immediate treatment
Rest. Ice. Ultrasound. Anti-inflammatory medication. Then heat and massage to promote blood flow and healing

Rehabilitation and prevention
Stretching the Achilles tendon and the plantar fascia will help speed recovery and prevent recurrence. A special orthotic or insert for the shoe may be required at the beginning of the return to activity. Strengthening the muscles of the lower leg will also serve to protect the fascia and prevent this condition.

Long-term prognosis
Most people with plantar fasciitis recover completely after a few weeks to a few months of treatment. Injections of corticosteroid may be necessary in cases where the fascia doesn't respond to early treatment.

HEEL SPUR

A heel spur is a hook or spike of bone on the calcaneus. Heel spurs are often associated with plantar fasciitis, although they may be seen without it. Spurs can occur on other bones as well.

When a section of bone becomes injured or irritated it will add calcium to the area to strengthen it. These calcium deposits become bone spurs. In the foot, heel spurs can form on the lower surface of the calcaneus, and sites where tendons or ligaments attach to bone are more commonly the sites of these spurs. Bone spurs irritate the tendons that cross over them, creating more inflammation within the tendon which may increase the spur.

Athletes with previous injuries or irritations of the tendon to bone attachments have a higher risk of bone spurs.

Cause of injury
Irritation of the plantar fascia at its calcaneal attachment. Untreated minor injury to bones. Calcium deposits on the outside of a healthy bone.

Signs and symptoms
Pain and tenderness at the heel. Possible grinding or clicking felt as the tendon crosses the spur.

Complications if left unattended
Bone spurs can cause injury to the tendons that pass over them which causes more inflammation and in turn may worsen the bone spur.

Immediate treatment
Rest from activities that cause pain. Anti-inflammatory medication.

Rehabilitation and prevention
Identifying and correcting the condition(s) that caused the irritation to the plantar fascia around the heel spur will help with recovery and prevent a recurrence of symptoms. Stretching the muscles and tendons involved will also speed recovery. The use of a heel cup, heel cradle or other orthotic device to reduce stress on the calcaneus may also help when returning to activity. Making sure to treat even minor injuries will also help prevent bone spurs.

Long-term prognosis
Heel spurs should respond well to rest and rehabilitation. Some may require orthotics to alleviate the symptoms and aid recovery. Surgery is occasionally required in individuals whose symptoms do not respond to conservative treatment.

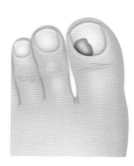

BLACK NAIL (SUBUNGUAL HAEMATOMA)

A subungual haematoma is bleeding under the toenail caused by an injury or infection to the nail bed. Crushing injury is the most common mechanism for this condition. The pocket of blood may be small or cover the whole area under the nail.

The nail protects the area under the toenail, the nail bed, but when crushing trauma, an object under the nail or infection causes damage to this soft area bleeding may occur. Because the nail is a hard surface it contains the bleeding which causes raised pressure in the nail bed and pain. Depending on the initial injury the underlying bone may also be involved.

Cause of injury
Crushing injury to the toe. Foreign object under the nail causing a laceration to the nail bed. Infection under the nail causing bleeding.

Signs and symptoms
Pain and pressure under the nail. Red, maroon or other dark colour under the nail.

Complications if left unattended
The bleeding and resulting pressure under the nail may cause damage to the underlying tissues causing necrosis over time. The nail may fall off and this could lead to infection if not treated properly. If the bone was fractured during the initial injury chronic pain may result.

Immediate treatment
Rest, ice and elevation. If the nail is lost it is important to keep the area covered and protected. If the possibility of a fracture exists, as with a crush injury, seek medical attention.

Rehabilitation and prevention
The nail may need to be removed during treatment, or may fall off on its own, leaving the nail bed exposed. It is important to keep this area protected to prevent infection. It is also important to protect the affected toe while it is healing. Padding over the toes may be needed. Avoiding impact to the toes and protecting them during activities will help prevent this injury.

Long-term prognosis
A subungual haematoma will usually respond well to treatment although in cases involving more than 25% of the nail bed and pressure that is unrelieved by initial treatments a physician may need to drain the blood from the nail bed. If an infection is the cause, oral or topical antibiotics may be required.

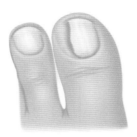

INGROWN TOENAIL

Ingrown (ingrowing) toenails can be very painful. They can result from trauma to the toe, tight-fitting shoes or improper grooming of the toenails. The toenail is a horny cutaneous plate which normally grows outward away from the base of the toe. It is made up of epithelial scales from the stratum lucidum of the skin. If the nail is cut or broken too close to the base it may grow into the skin on the side of the toe, or the skin may grow over the toenail.

Injury to the toe, such as stubbing the toe or a toe fracture, can cause the toenail to grow into the skin. Tight-fitting shoes may also put pressure on the outside of the toe pressing skin into the nail and causing it to grow over the nail. Pain and infection may also result from the skin growing over the nail or the nail growing into the skin on the sides. Redness and swelling on the outside of the toe may also be noted.

Cause of injury
Trauma to the toe, such as stubbing the toe. Tight or improperly fitting shoes. Improper toenail grooming.

Signs and symptoms
Pain. Redness and swelling in the affected area. Pus or other signs of infection may be present.

Complications if left unattended
If left unattended an ingrown toenail may become infected and the infection may eventually involve the entire toe or even the foot. The pain may become chronic and affect the ability to wear certain shoes. The athlete may develop a limp.

Immediate treatment
Soak the foot in warm water. Get rid of tight-fitting shoes and select roomier ones. Keep the feet dry during the day. Seek the assistance of a qualified podiatrist.

Rehabilitation and prevention
When treating an ingrown nail it is important to protect it from additional trauma or injury. Change socks as needed to keep the feet dry. Wearing shoes with plenty of room for the toes will aid healing and prevent further ingrown toenails. Protecting the toes from trauma will also help prevent this condition. After trauma to the toe it is important to check the toenails for breakage and pressing of the nail into the skin.

Long-term prognosis
Ingrown toenails commonly respond to treatment and repair completely. Ingrown toenails may become a recurring problem in some cases, especially if the underlying causes are not addressed. In cases where infection has set in and does not respond to initial treatment surgery may be required. Removal of all or part of the toenail and the infected tissue may be required.

REHABILITATION EXERCISES

Bounding

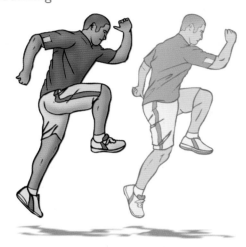

In a running motion, raise one knee and jump upward and forward propelling off your back foot. Continue running forward with an exaggerated high arm action.

Zigzag shuffle

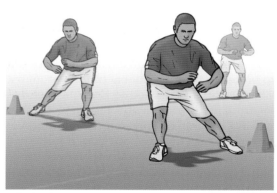

While keeping your body facing forward, push outward with your feet as you run sideways from one cone to the next.

Calf muscle stretch – soleus

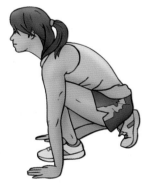

Stand upright while leaning against a wall and place one foot behind the other. Make sure that both toes are facing forward and your heel is on the ground. Bend your back leg and lean toward the wall.

Foot stretch

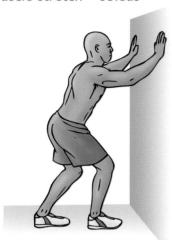

Kneel on one foot with your hands on the ground. Place your body weight over your knee and slowly move your knee forward. Keep your toes on the ground and arch your foot.

Glossary of Terms

Abrasion. Skin wound in which the external layers have been rubbed/scraped off.

Achilles tendinitis. Inflammation of the Achilles tendon.

Acute injury. Injury from a specific event leading to a sudden onset of symptoms.

Adhesive capsulitis. Adhesive inflammation between the joint capsule and the peripheral articular cartilage of the glenohumeral joint in the shoulder. Causes pain, stiffness and limitation of movement. Also known as frozen shoulder.

Anterior tibial compartment syndrome. Swelling, tightness and pain of the anterior tibial compartment of the leg. Usually a history of excessive exertion.

Arthropathy. Any joint disease.

Atrophy. Wasting or deterioration of tissue due to disease, disuse or malnutrition.

Articular dysfunction. Disturbance, impairment or abnormality of a joint.

Avulsion fracture. Fracture where a bone fragment becomes separated from the main bone at the sight of tendinous attachments, often due to excessive tensile forces.

Baker's cyst. Swelling behind the knee, caused by leakage of synovial fluid into the popliteal bursa.

Blister. Fluid accumulation under the skin caused by friction of the skin against a hard or rough surface causing the epidermis to separate from the dermis.

Bunion. Swelling over the medial aspect of the first metatarsophalangeal joint resulting in displacement of the great toe (hallux valgus).

Bursa. Protective sac containing synovial fluid, typically found between tendons and bones. It acts to reduce friction during movement.

Bursitis. Inflammation of a bursa, e.g. subacromial bursitis.

Calcific tendinitis. Inflammation and calcification of the muscle tendon. Most commonly seen in the rotator cuff of the shoulder.

Callus. Localized thickening of epidermis due to physical trauma.

Cancellous. Bone tissue of relatively low density.

Capsulitis. Inflammation of a joint capsule.

Carpal tunnel syndrome. Compression of the median nerve as it passes through the carpal tunnel, leading to pain and tingling in the hand.

Cauliflower ear. Haematoma between the perichondrium and cartilage of the outer ear.

Chondral fracture. Fracture involving the articular cartilage of a joint.

Chondromalacia patellae. Degenerative condition in the articular cartilage of the patella caused by abnormal compression or shearing forces.

Chronic injury. Injury characterized by a slow, sustained development of symptoms that culminates in a painful inflammatory condition.

Claw toe. Toe deformity, particularly in patients with rheumatoid arthritis, consisting of dorsal subluxation of toes 2–5; painful condition during walking. The patient develops a shuffling gait.

Collateral ligaments. Major ligaments that cross the medial and lateral aspects of a joint.

Colles' fracture. Fracture of the radius and ulna, just proximal to the wrist, that results in the distal segment displacing in a dorsal and radial direction.

Compressive force. Axial loading that produces a squeezing effect on a structure.

Compartment syndrome. Condition in which increased intramuscular pressure impedes blood flow and function of tissues within the fascial compartment.

Concussion. Violent shaking or jarring of the brain resulting in immediate or transient impairment of neurological function.

Contracture. Adhesion formation in an immobilized muscle, leading to a shortened contractile state.

Contraindication. A condition adversely affected by a specific action.

Contusion. Compression injury involving accumulation of blood and lymph within a muscle. Also known as a bruise.

Cruciate ligaments. Major ligaments that criss-cross the knee in the anteroposterior direction.

Deep vein thrombosis (DVT). The formation of a stationary blood clot in the wall of one or more of the deep veins of the lower leg.

De Quervain's tenosynovitis. Inflammatory tenosynovitis of the abductor pollicis longus and extensor pollicis brevis tendons in the thumb.

Diffuse injury. Injury over a large body area, usually due to low-velocity/high-mass forces.

Discogenic pain. Pain caused by derangement of an intervertebral disc.

Discopathy. Disease of an intervertebral disc.

Efferent nerves. Nerves carrying stimuli from the central nervous system.

Epicondylitis. Inflammation and traction apophysitis on the epicondyles of the distal humerus.

Epiphyseal fracture. Injury to the growth plate of a long bone in children and adolescents; may lead to arrested bone growth.

Erythema. Redness of the skin produced by congestion of the capillaries.

Fasciitis. Inflammation of the fascial envelopes surrounding muscles.

Fracture. A disruption in the continuity of a bone.

Frozen shoulder. See adhesive capsulitis.

Ganglion cyst. Benign mass commonly seen on the dorsal aspect of the wrist.

Golfer's elbow. Inflammation of periosteum at the medial epicondyle of the humerus caused by activities (e.g. golf) that involve gripping, flexion and pronation of the forearm.

Haematoma. Localized mass of blood and lymph confined within a space or tissue.

Hallux. The first, or great, toe.

Hallux rigidus. Painful flexion deformity of the great toe in which there is limitation of motion at the metatarsophalangeal joint.

Hallux valgus. Angulation of the great toe toward the second toe.

Hammer toe. Hyperextension/flexion deformity of the toes.

Heel spur. Bony spur formation on the calcaneus.

Hernia. Protrusion of abdominal viscera through a weakened portion of the abdominal wall.

Herniated disc. Rupture of an intervertebral disc causing the inner content to push out.

Hip pointer. Contusions caused by direct compression to an unprotected iliac crest that crushes soft tissue and, sometimes, the bone itself.

Iliotibial band syndrome. Pain/inflammation at the iliotibial band, a tough, fibrous thickening of the fascia of the lower limb stretching from the iliac crest of the hip to below the knee. There are various biomechanical causes.

Impingement syndrome. Chronic shoulder condition caused by repetitive overhead activity that damages the glenoid labrum, long head of biceps brachii and the subacromial bursa.

Inflammation. Protective response to tissue damage characterized by pain, swelling, redness, heat and loss of function.

Innervation. Nerve supply of a tissue.

Ischaemia. Local oxygen deficiency due to decreased blood supply.

Laceration. Wound that may leave a smooth or jagged edge through the skin, subcutaneous tissues, muscles and associated nerves and blood vessels.

Larson-Johansson syndrome. Inflammation or partial avulsion of the apex of the patella due to traction forces.

Lesion. Any pathological or traumatic discontinuity of tissue or loss of function of a part.

Lordosis. The concave curve in the lumbar region of the spine.

Mallet finger. Rupture of the extensor tendon from the distal phalanx due to forceful flexion of the phalanx.

Menisci. Fibrocartilage discs within the knee that reduce joint stress.

Meralgia paraesthetica. Entrapment of the lateral femoral cutaneous nerve at the inguinal ligament, causing pain and numbness of the outer surface of the thigh in the region supplied by the nerve.

Metatarsalgia. Pain around the metatarsal heads in the foot.

Microtrauma. Small-scale injury to the tissues of the musculoskeletal system.

Morton's neuralgia. Pain around the metatarsals caused by compression of a branch of the plantar nerve by the metatarsal heads.

Morton's neuroma. Thickening and fibrosis causing compression of the plantar nerve in the foot, resulting in Morton's neuralgia.

Muscle spindle. Encapsulated receptor sensitive to stretch found in muscle tissue.

Myositis. Inflammation of connective tissues within a muscle.

Myositis ossificans. Accumulation of calcium deposits in muscle tissue.

Neuritis. Inflammation of a nerve.

Neuropathy. Functional disturbance or pathological change in a nerve.

Non-union fracture. A fracture in which healing is delayed or fails to unite.

NSAID. Non-steroidal anti-inflammatory drug.

Oedema. Accumulation of lymphatic fluid in the tissues caused by failure of the lymphatic system to drain properly.

Osgood-Schlatter disease. Inflammation or partial avulsion of the patellar ligament at the tibial apophysis due to traction forces.

Osteitis. Inflammation of a bone, causing enlargement of the bone, tenderness and dull, aching pain.

Osteoarthritis. Non-inflammatory degenerative joint disease characterized by degeneration of the articular cartilage, hypertrophy of bone at the margins and changes in the synovial membrane. Seen particularly in older persons.

Osteochondritis dissecans. Localized area of avascular necrosis resulting from complete or incomplete separation of joint cartilage and subchondral bone.

Overuse injury. Any injury caused by excessive, repetitive movement of the body part.

Painful arc syndrome. Shoulder pain on abduction (elevation) of the arm from 60–120 degrees.

Paralysis. Partial or complete loss of the ability to move a body part.

Passive stretching. Stretching of muscles, tendons and ligaments produced by a stretching force other than tension in the antagonist muscles.

Patellofemoral stress syndrome. A painful condition where the lateral patella retinaculum is tight or the vastus medialis muscle is weak, leading to lateral excursion and pressure on the lateral facet of the patella.

Pes cavus. Abnormally high medial arch of the foot.

Pes planus. Flat feet or fallen arches (may be flexible or rigid).

Plantar fascia. Specialized band of fascia that covers the plantar surface of the foot and helps support the longitudinal arch.

Plyometric training. Exercises that employ explosive movements to develop muscular power.

Posterior compartment syndrome. Pain and reduced function due to raised pressure causing compression of vessels in the posterior fascial compartments of the lower leg.

Prognosis. Prediction of the likely progress or outcome of an injury.

Proprioceptors. Specialized deep sensory nerve cells in joints, ligaments, muscles and tendons sensitive to stretch, tension and pressure which are responsible for joint and limb position sense.

Q-angle. Angle between the line of quadriceps force and the patellar (tendon) ligament.

Radiculopathy. Disease of spinal nerve roots.
Referred pain. Pain felt in a region of the body other than where the source or cause of the pain is located.
Repetitive strain injury (RSI). Refers to any overuse condition such as strain or tendonitis in any part of the body.
Rheumatoid arthritis. Autoimmune disease in which the immune system attacks the body's own tissues. Causes inflammation of many parts of the body and damage to synovial joints.
Rotator cuff. The SITS (supraspinatus, infraspinatus, teres minor, and subscapularis) muscles that hold the head of the humerus in the glenoid fossa and produce humeral rotation.

Sacroiliitis. Inflammation of the sacroiliac joint.
Scapulocostal syndrome. Pain in the superior or posterior aspect of the shoulder girdle as a result of long-standing alteration of the relationship between the scapula and the posterior thoracic wall.
Sciatica. Pain in the distribution of the sciatic nerve due to a herniated disc, a muscle-related or facet joint disease or compression by piriformis.
Scoliosis. Lateral rotational spinal curvature.
Seronegative spondyloarthropathy. A group of inflammatory rheumatic diseases causing synovitis of peripheral joints.
Sesamoid bones. Small bones embedded in tendons – the largest is the patella.
Sesamoiditis. Inflammation of the sesamoid bones of the first metatarsal.
Sever's disease. A traction-type injury or osteochondrosis of the calcaneal apophysis seen in young adolescents.
Shear force. A force that acts parallel or tangentially to a plane passing through an object.
Snapping hip syndrome. A snapping sensation either heard or felt during motion at the hip.
Somatic pain. Pain originating in the skin, ligaments, muscles, bones or joints.
Spasm. Transitory muscle contractions.
Spondyloarthropathy. Disease of the joints of the spine.
Spondylolisthesis. Forward displacement of one vertebra over another.
Spondylolysis. Fracture of a vertebra (usually at the vertebral arch).
Spondylosis. Degenerative spinal changes due to osteoarthritis.
Sprain. Injury to ligamentous tissue.
Static stretch. Slow, sustained muscle stretching used to increase flexibility.
Stenosis. Abnormal narrowing of a duct or canal, e.g. spinal stenosis, a narrowing of the vertebral canal, caused by encroachment of the bone upon the space.
Strain. Injury to muscle or ligamentous tissue.
Stress. The distribution of force within a body.
Stress (march) fracture. Hairline crack of a bone caused by excessive repetitive stress.
Subungual haematoma. Collection of blood under the nail.
Synovitis. Inflammation of a synovial membrane, particularly of a joint.

Tendinopathy. Disease of a tendon.
Tendinitis. Inflammation of a tendon. Also known as tendonitis.
Tennis elbow. Tendinitis of the extensor muscles of the forearm at their insertion on the lateral epicondyle of the humerus. Also known as lateral epicondylitis.

Tenosynovitis. Inflammation of a tendon sheath.

Resources

Anderson, D.M. (chief lexicographer): 2003. *Dorland's Illustrated Medical Dictionary, 30th edition*. Saunders, an imprint of Elsevier, Philadelphia
Anderson, M.K. & Hall, S.J.: 1997. *Fundamentals of Sports Injury Management*. Williams & Wilkins, Baltimore
Arnheim, D.D.: 1989. *Modern Principles of Athletic Training*. Times Mirror, MO
Bahr, R. & Maehlum, S.: 2004. *Clinical Guide to Sports Injuries*. Human Kinetics, Champaign
Cramer, J.T., Housh, T.J., Weir, J.P., Johnson, G.O., Coburn, J.W. and Beck, T.W.: 2005. *The acute effects of static stretching on peak torque, mean power output, electromyography, and mechanomyography*. European Journal of Applied Psychology. Vol. 93: 5–6, 530-539
Delavier, F.: 2001. *Strength Training Anatomy*. Human Kinetics, Champaign
Dornan, P. & Dunn, R.: 1988. *Sporting Injuries*. University of Queensland Press, Queensland
Jarmey, C.: 2008. *The Concise Book of Muscles, 2nd edition*. Lotus Publishing, Chichester
Jarmey, C.: 2006. *The Concise Book of the Moving Body*. Lotus Publishing, Chichester
Klossner, D.: 2006. *NCAA Sports Medicine Handbook*. The National Collegiate Athletic Association, IN
Lamb, D.R.: 1984. *Physiology of Exercise*. Macmillan Publishing Co., New York
Levy, A.M. & Fuerst, M.L.: 1993. *Sports Injury Handbook*. John Wiley & Sons, Inc., New York
Micheli, L.J.: 1995. *Sports Medicine Bible*. HarperCollins Publishers, Inc., New York
Norris, C.M.: 1998. *Sports Injuries: Diagnosis and Management*. Butterworth Heinemann, Oxford,
Reid, M.G.: 1994. *Sports Medicine Awareness Course*. Sports Medicine Federation, ACT, Australia
Rushall, B.S. & Pyke, F.S.: 1990. *Training for Sports and Fitness*. Macmillan Education Australia, New South Wales
Sports Medicine Australia: 1986. *The Sports Trainer*. Jacaranda Press, Queensland
Tortora, G.J. & Anagnostakos, N.P.: 1990. *Principles of Anatomy and Physiology*. Harper & Row, New York
United States Consumer Product Safety Commission: 2000. *Consumer Product Safety Review. Spring, Vol. 4: 4*
Walker, B.E.: 1998. *The Stretching Handbook*. Walkerbout Health, Robina
Walker, B.E.: 2006. *The Sports Injury Handbook*. Walkerbout Health, Robina
Walker, B.E.: 2011. *The Anatomy of Stretching, 2nd edition*. Lotus Publishing, Chichester

Index